Confronting the Malpractice Crisis

Guidelines for the Obstetrician-Gynecologist

edited by

Daniel K. Roberts

M.D., Ph.D., F.A.C.O.G.

Jeffrey A. Shane

M.D., J.D., F.A.C.O.G.

Margaret L. Roberts

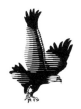

Eagle Press

Kansas City

Library of Congress Cataloging in Publication Data

Main entry under title:

Confronting the malpractice crisis.

    Includes bibliographies and index.
    1. Obstetricians—Malpractice—United States.
2. Gynecologists—Malpractice—United States.
3. Forensic obstetrics.   4. Forensic gynecology.
I. Roberts, Daniel K.   II. Shane, Jeffrey A.
III. Roberts, Margaret L.   [DNLM: 1. Financial
Management—methods.   2. Gynecology—United States—
legislation.   3. Malpractice—United States—legislation.
4. Obstetrics—United States—legislation.   WQ 33 AA1 C7]
KF2910.G943C66 1985   346.7303'32   85-10187
ISBN 0-935868-12-7   347.306332

ISBN 0-935868-12-7

Eagle Press
Post Office Box 2404
Kansas City, Kansas 66110

Acknowledgments

This book owes its being to the dedicated efforts of many people. Besides our heartfelt gratitude to those who wrote chapters, we wish to acknowledge the excellent contributions made by Cathy S. Biggs, Montie R. Deer, Ruth M. Smith, and Patricia E. Summers. We also want to gratefully thank the staff and residents of the Department of Obstetrics and Gynecology at Wesley Medical Center, University of Kansas School of Medicine–Wichita, for their encouragement and support.

Table of Contents

Reviewing the Crisis

Understanding the Law

Managing the Risk

Entering the Future

Appendixes

Contributors

John A. Anderson, M.D., J.D.

Colonel, United States Air Force; Commander, United States Air Force Hospital Beale, Beale Air Force Base, California; Assistant Clinical Professor of Radiology, University of California–Davis College of Medicine, Davis, California; Diplomate, American Board of Law in Medicine; Diplomate, American Board of Radiology; Fellow, American College of Legal Medicine; Member, American College of Physician Executives.

George J. Annas, J.D.

Edward Utley Professor of Health Law, Boston University Schools of Medicine and Public Health, Boston, Massachusetts; Chairman, Legal Problems in Medicine Committee, Science and Technology Section, American Bar Association.

David P. Calvert, J.D.

Partner, Curfman, Harris, Stallings, and Snow, Wichita, Kansas. Formerly, Judge, District Court, Division 9, 18th Judicial District of Kansas, Wichita, Kansas.

Sherman Elias, M.D.

Director, Medical Genetic Services, Prentice Women's Hospital and Maternity Center; Associate Professor of Obstetrics and Gynecology, Northwestern University Medical School, Chicago, Illinois.

Charles M. Jacobs, J.D.

Chairman and Chief Executive Officer, MediQual Systems, Inc., Westborough, Massachusetts; President, InterQual, Incorporated, Chicago, Illinois; Of Counsel, Siegan, Barbakoff, Gomberg, Gordon, and Elden, Limited, Chicago, Illinois. Formerly, Associate Director, Joint Commission on Accreditation of Hospitals.

Walter A. Oleniewski, J.D., M.F.S.

Principal, Joling, Rizzo, Willems, Oleniewski, and Burroughs, S.C., Kenosha, Wisconsin. Formerly, Assistant Director, Torts Branch, Civil Division, United States Department of Justice, Washington, D.C.

Elvoy Raines, J.D.

Associate Executive Director, American Society of Law and Medicine; Doctoral Candidate, Harvard School of Public Health, Department of Health Policy and Management, Boston, Massachusetts. Formerly, Associate Director, Professional Liability; Associate Director, Government Relations, American College of Obstetricians and Gynecologists, Washington, D.C.

Edgar A. Reed, M.D., J.D.

Chief of Staff, Veterans Administration Medical Center, Livermore, California; Fellow and Board of Governors, American College of Legal Medicine; Editor, Legal Aspects of Medical Practice; Associate Clinical Professor, University of California at Davis. Formerly, Director, Medical-Legal Affairs, Veterans Administration, Washington, D.C.; Chairman, American Board of Law in Medicine, 1981–1984; President, American College of Legal Medicine, 1981–1982; President, Medical-Legal Associates, Incorporated.

Daniel K. Roberts, M.D., Ph.D.

Chairman and Professor, Department of Obstetrics and Gynecology; Professor, Department of Pathology, University of Kansas School of Medicine–Wichita, Wichita, Kansas; Fellow, American College of Obstetricians and Gynecologists.

Margaret L. Roberts

President, Medical-Legal Consultants, Incorporated, Wichita, Kansas.

Jeffrey A. Shane, M.D., J.D.

Attorney, Shulman, Rogers, Gandal, Tobin, and Ecker, P.A., Silver Spring, Maryland; Fellow, American College of Obstetricians and Gynecologists; Fellow, American College of Legal Medicine. Formerly, Chief, Division of Medical-Legal Consultation, Department of Legal Medicine, Armed Forces Institute of Pathology, Washington, D.C.

James G. Zimmerly, M.D., J.D., M.P.H.

Chairman, Department of Legal Medicine, Armed Forces Institute of Pathology, Washington, D.C.; Editor, Lawyer's Medical Cyclopedia; Editor, Maryland Medical Journal; Adjunct Professor, Georgetown University Law Center; Associate Professor, University of Maryland School of Medicine. Formerly, President, American College of Legal Medicine.

Preface

Obstetricians are currently the megabuck targets of many lawsuits. Gynecologists are not far behind. The results of a questionnaire distributed in 1980 to all section chairmen of the American College of Obstetricians and Gynecologists (ACOG) revealed that malpractice was the number two concern of the Fellows.* There is little doubt that medical malpractice is again the focus of a crisis that will far exceed that of the mid-1970s. This earlier crisis was primarily one of unavailability of insurance or, at least, its unavailability at a reasonable cost. Numerous sociolegislative adjustments reduced the status of the crisis to one of quiescent plateau. The combination of the publicity surrounding the problem, the new legislation passed, and the uncertain effect of the latter maintained this plateau from 1976 until early 1979 when a sudden increase in litigation began. As this new crisis has surged, obstetricians and gynecologists have risen to the top of the legal hit list.

Obstetricians and gynecologists, as well as other physicians, are an interesting Pavlovian breed. When personally touched by a stimulus, they respond vigorously. When the stimulus is removed, complacency sets in. During the mid-1970s, many were ready to do anything they could to resolve the crisis. However, bandaids made these same individuals complacent. The ACOG questionnaire indicated an obvious return of interest.

In the collective experience of the contributors to this book, we have found that major problems in appropriately responding to litigation are directly attributable to the physician's lack of understanding of the

---

* Stone, ML. Personal communication, 1981.

legal process. Fear of the unknown has time and again had a major negative influence on the outcome of a case that would have otherwise been resolved in favor of the defendant-physician. Here is a simple illustration.

> A very competent obstetrician-gynecologist had successfully completed a vaginal hysterectomy using standard operative technique. On the third postoperative day, the patient developed a vaginal cuff infection which was recognized and treated appropriately. Nevertheless, a pinpoint rectal-vaginal fistula occurred which caused the patient little difficulty and was successfully repaired three months later. The patient filed suit for alleged negligence in performing the original procedure and lack of informed consent. The plaintiff's attorney readily admitted that after talking to his medical expert he was ready to advise his client that there was insufficient cause to continue the case. However, in closely reviewing the records, he found that because of fear and ignorance of the common law regarding informed consent in that state, the physician had squeezed in, after the fact, a one-line reference to informed consent regarding infection and possible fistula. With this act alone, the physician destroyed his own credibility, and his insurance company paid out $75,000 in an otherwise nonmeritorious case.

We do not believe that knowledge and familiarity with the legal process will successfully remove all malpractice litigation. The most competent physicians occasionally deviate from the standard of good medical practice; and if this deviation results in an injury, the plaintiff may successfully recover damages. We do believe, however, that adequate knowledge and familiarity with the legal system will:

- remove the fear of the unknown;
- allow a thorough appraisal of the case with an appropriate evaluation of its merit or relative merit;
- allow appropriate, early, and continued physician involvement in the process;
- bring about more appropriate and, perhaps, smaller settlements for meritorious cases;
- result more often in the successful defense of nonmeritorious or borderline cases;
- reduce the overall cost to the whole health care system; and
- ultimately create an equitable system for both patient and physician alike.

To begin to approach these goals, the contributors to this text describe the legal system, give case examples, and offer helpful guidelines in the management of litigious problems. However, although the authors address the fundamentals of the malpractice problem, the book is not intended to provide counsel for individual or specific cases or situations that necessarily should be provided by personal counsel. In addition, because of the differences in law from jurisdiction to jurisdiction, legal questions about a particular circumstance should be referred to a local attorney who can apply specific state holdings.

No work on such a topic would be complete without a couple of additional obligatory disclaimers. First, opinions expressed in the individual chapters are those of the authors themselves and do not necessarily represent the opinions of either the editors or the publisher. Second, while suggestions and recommendations may be helpful in decreasing the frequency of lawsuits, no one could or would with any certainty suggest that any action is guaranteed to either prevent a lawsuit from being brought or predict what the outcome in a case might be. Surefire cures for the malpractice crisis are like surefire cures for disease; they do not exist now and they probably will not exist in the future.

One additional caveat—law and medicine are both dynamic areas of human interaction, and the interface between them presents a rapidly changing, multifaceted, kaleidoscopic picture that must be frozen in time to put down on paper. In other words, we had to choose a cutoff date for updating the material.

Let us conclude with a look back and a look forward. From prehistoric times, those entrusted with the knowledge of healing have been afforded a special respect—but this respect has always demanded accountability. Since the twelfth century, the accountability of medical professionals has been defined and administered by the legal system. However, in the past four decades, medicine has made a quantum leap forward, and the law's response has often been confusing and contradictory. We examine the recent circumstances that have produced an escalating medical liability crisis; we address how to deal with these issues on a day-to-day basis; and we explore what lies ahead for the resolution of this ongoing dilemma. These are subjects that demand our attention.

Daniel K. Roberts
Jeffrey A. Shane
Margaret L. Roberts

Reviewing the Crisis

In the mid-1970s, the medical profession and the country were shocked by what has universally been called the medical malpractice crisis. We define this earlier crisis, examine the circumstances that precipitated it, and explore the solutions that were attempted. Since resolution has not occurred and a new crisis is already at hand, reviewing the crisis of the mid-1970s and observing the results may guide us toward meaningful solutions.

1

Chapter 1

Malpractice in Perspective

Daniel K. Roberts

Although many of us believe that malpractice is one of those black clouds that began when we graduated from medical school and has followed us ever since, history tells us otherwise. The first medical negligence case was recorded in England in 1374, and the first American case was in Connecticut in 1794.[1] Adding to this historical perspective is the following excerpt from a book published in 1932 by Lloyd Paul Stryker, who was for many years the general counsel for the New York Medical Society.[2]

> But it is another ill of the medical profession,—an ill having grave economic possibilities—which is the occasion of this book—an ill which is due both to a public misunderstanding of the medical profession and the unscrupulousness of certain types of patients. I refer, of course, to the increasing frequency with which doctors are being sued for malpractice. This evil is not new. More than half a century ago Dr. Oliver Wendell Holmes was writing that 'the profession has just been startled by a verdict against a physician ruinous in its amount,—enough to drive many a hard working young practitioner out of house and home—a verdict which leads to the fear that suits for malpractice may take the place of the panel game and child stealing as a means of extorting money. If the profession in this state, which claims a high standard of civilization, is to be crushed and ground beneath the upper millstone of the dearth of educational advantages and the lower millstone of ruinous penalties for what the *ignorant ignorantly shall decide to be ignorance,* all I can say is, "God save the Commonwealth of Massachusetts"' [p. xxiii, emphasis added].

Although these comments by Dr. Holmes were made in the late 1800s, they are not far from the attitude of many modernday physicians. The contributors to this volume present a more reasoned approach—some malpractice actions are reasonable and justified and some are not; physicians cannot play ostrich to either category. For the sake of our patients, we should educate ourselves and our colleagues to assure the best of medical care, to discipline bad practitioners when necessary, and to testify in justifiable cases. For the sake of our profession, we should vigorously support and defend reasonable practitioners against frivolous, malicious, and unwarranted actions.

In 1970, one in twenty-five physicians was sued.[3] Yet, the statistics were similar in 1932 when Stryker noted:

> The membership of the Medical Society of the State of New York is approximately 12,500 physicians. In 1930 there were 256 more malpractice suits brought against members of the Medical Society of the State of New York than in 1929, a thirty-three per cent increase, and representing one suit for malpractice for every twenty-two members of the Society [p. vii].

While I do not intend to suggest that things were no worse in 1970 than in 1932, I do want to emphasize that malpractice litigation is a continuing reality in the daily practice of medicine. However, current statistics indicate a radical departure from this trend; in the years following 1970, one in ten physicians were sued, some resulting in eight digit, megabuck awards.[4] Whether or not these crisis proportions continue throughout the foreseeable future, there is currently sufficient litigious activity to suggest that physicians must learn how to cope with it and how to counteract its unfair aspects. In other words, we must be knowledgeable not only in the practice of medicine but, to some degree, in the applications of tort law.

While there is no way to accurately assess the extent of actual malpractice, most medical practitioners have felt for some time that too many patients and their attorneys erroneously equate bad outcomes or maloccurrences with malpractice. Physicians know that there are many mistakes and deviations from the standard of good medical practice that do not result in injury; further, many injuries are complications that are not the result of negligent acts or omisssions by medical personnel. However, as Mills illustrates in the California Medical Insurance Feasibility Study,* the adversarial battleground exists between the "in-

---

* See Appendix B for a detailed summary of this study.

cidence of medically caused patient disabilities" and "the incidence of legal fault by members of the health care professions" (p. 2).[5]

Malpractice litigation is a matter of civil law and more specifically tort law or law of injury. The physician is accused of either doing something that should not have been done by a reasonable and prudent physician under the same or similar circumstances (comission) or of not doing something that a reasonable and prudent physician would have done under the same or similar conditions (omission), i.e., whether or not there was a deviation from the standard of good medical practice. Under our legal system, a jury decides whether such a deviation occurred and, if so, whether it was the proximate cause of the injury. Both the accused physician and the injured patient are offered the opportunity to educate a lay jury regarding their respective positions. Without prior education and/or background, the jury makes decisions that are based on the crash course provided by litigants. In spite of whatever evidence is presented, these decisions cannot help but be based on a foundation of ignorance.

A portion of the fault lies in the lack of communication between physicians and attorneys, which encourages stereotypes, endangers cooperation, and fosters misunderstanding. For example, the medical community tends to feel that physicians put up the stakes and the lawyers roll the dice, that they are the big players since the plaintiff's lawyer has the potential big jackpot and the defense lawyer collects his hourly wage throughout the slow and grueling legal process. Lawyers and physicians are both professionals, and it is no more true that all lawyers are shysters than it is that all physicians are incompetents.

Though both are professionals, they differ. The doctor's

education, while prolonged and intensive, is rather structured and narrow. It is primarily scientific in scope. He is taught to measure, to observe and, above all, *to be objective*. He becomes a specialist the day he enters medical school; a specialist in the art and science of medicine.

In a way, a set of blinders is put on him at the outset. In the environment in which he leads his professional life, other people wait upon him. His authority and knowledge are rarely questioned. He is resentful if they are. Every day he must make decisions that can have far-reaching effects upon the lives of his patients; he often must make those decisions immediately [and frequently with incomplete data]. Usually, his work totally consumes his available time and energy. He is not much given to philosophical meditation.

But, headiest of all, is the total control he has over those patients who come to him. Life, health and well-being are things people value greatly, and they entrust them all to the doctor. Is it any wonder that he sometimes develops a sort of 'God complex'? It is a difficult thing to resist or even avoid. In time, this can make the admission of fallibility very awkward indeed [p. 33].[6]

But what of the lawyer? Physicians need to understand that

the lawyer, and in particular the trial lawyer, is a different man. His education is not the same at all; it is much broader. He deals with words, their use and interpretation. He deals with abstractions. He is trained to probe, question, and analyze. He searches for any area, fact or interpretation of fact, relevant or irrelevant, with only one thing in mind: his aim is to win. He does not actually concern himself about the rightness or wrongness of an issue. His concern is to settle a dispute, to settle it as advantageously as he can for himself and his client but, above all, to settle it. He is the adversary in a war and cannot comprehend that the doctor does not view his effort as proper.

But, this concept of war is completely foreign to the doctor. The doctor, by training and expectation, seeks truth. The lawyer knows that absolute truth is rarely, if ever, found and is satisfied to look for *probability* [p. 33].[6]

To fully appreciate the difference between these two professions, we medical practitioners must educate ourselves. We must understand attorneys and the tactics they use, which will enable us to assist in our defense or to contribute as expert witnesses. In fact, the more understanding we have of the legal system in general, the less fearful we are and the greater assets we become. This book was written to give those in the health care professions an introduction to the legal process as well as some guidelines for precluding litigation.

References

1. Stetler, CJ. The history of reported medical professional liability cases. Temple Law Q 30(4):366, 1957.
2. Stryker, LP. Courts and doctors. New York: Macmillan, 1932.
3. Jacobs, CM. Hospital risk management and malpractice liability control. Chicago: InterQual, 1980.
4. Danzon, PM. The frequency and severity of medical malpractice claims. Santa Monica, CA: Rand Corporation, 1983.
5. Mills, DH, ed. Report on the medical insurance feasibility study. San Francisco: California Medical Association, 1977.
6. Frink, NW. "The twain must meet or . . . ." Trial 11(3):32, 1975.

Chapter 2

The Crisis of the Mid-1970s in Review

Charles M. Jacobs and Daniel K. Roberts

Beginning in the fall of 1974 and continuing for over a year, a crisis existed in the medical malpractice arena. The precipitating factor of this crisis was not increased medical malpractice activity, but rather the unprecedented climb in malpractice insurance premiums. Across the nation, insurance premiums had jumped precipitously; and in some areas, insurance was not available at any price. The nation faced disruption in medical services because of the unavailability of professional liability insurance. Scattered doctors' strikes and pleas from many sectors for legislative action brought attention to the crisis.

By the fall of 1976, although the frequency and cost of malpractice claims were growing at an alarming rate, the crisis precipitated by the unavailability of malpractice insurance seemed to have disappeared. Insurance companies offered coverage through a variety of mechanisms, though at higher premiums. What happened in the two years between crisis and resolution is instructive. James K. Cooper and Sharman Stephens of the Department of Health, Education, and Welfare (DHEW) closely monitored the events of those two years and developed an excellent analysis of the crisis and its causative factors.[1]

Prior to the crisis and in spite of the January 1973 DHEW report to the contrary, scattered reports surfaced that malpractice insurance was in danger of no longer being available. Two years later, in the fall of 1974, seven states indicated that major insurance carriers were withdrawing from the market and that smaller companies expressed little or no interest in providing coverage. Of twenty-two commercial carriers providing insurance in 1971, only seven were doing so by 1976. Those insurance companies that continued to offer coverage requested state insurance commissioners to approve general rate increases of 100 percent, then 200 percent in New York and 300 percent in California. Premiums for the highest risk subspecialists (e.g., neurosurgeons, plastic surgeons) increased as much as 750 percent, approaching $50,000 for $1 million/$3 million coverage.[2] Increased insurance rates also affected hospitals, causing their premiums to escalate 200 to 300 percent and amounting to more than one million dollars per year in some instances.

Causes of the Medical Malpractice Crisis in the Mid-1970s

Claims-Related Causes

The withdrawal of many insurance carriers from the market and the enormous rate increases by those companies that remained caused the crisis. These decisions were based on the escalating frequency (number of claims) and the increasing severity (amount of awards to injured plaintiffs) that made it impossible to predict the risk to be underwritten. For example, between 1967 and 1973, the frequency and severity of claims increased ten to twelve percent per year.

While the increasing frequency and severity of claims was the primary cause of the crisis in insurance availability, other factors affected the insurance industry, exacerbating the problem of predicting the risk to be underwritten. First, the magnitude of the annual increases was largely unforeseen. Although careful retrospective analysis of the trends in tort law and of claims data from 1970 to 1972 can be used to argue that the crisis was predictable, no scholar, legal commentator, or, most importantly, insurance actuary envisioned the magnitude of what was to come.

The ability to predict trends in medical malpractice claim losses is complicated by the unique characteristic of the so-called *long tail.* The tail is the time lag between the occurrence of an injury and the settlement or closing of a claim. For medical malpractice, the average tail may be several times that of other types of liability. For example, while half of all automobile injury claims are settled within six months, half of all medical malpractice claims are not settled until two years or more following the incident.

Second, little data existed in 1974 and 1975 that adequately described the financial aspects of the malpractice insurance industry or the nature of the risk being undertaken. In this time period, no data outside the insurance industry identified the profitability of medical malpractice insurance as a separate line of insurance; in fact, occasionally insurers stated that professional liability insurance was a "loss leader," sold in order to capture a lucrative market for other high profit insurance. Since premiums were relatively inexpensive prior to 1974, physicians did not demand data supporting premium rates; and state insurance commissioners, whose duty was to approve rates, had no specific need for the data. The data available at the time provided only general information regarding profiles of defendants, characteristics of injuries, and sites of injury. In fact, physicians viewed malpractice suits like rain that fell equally on the competent and the incompetent—perhaps more on competent physicians because they undertook the more difficult cases. Inability to predict the risk of loss caused the crisis in insurance availability. Other insurance industry factors, such as the shrinkage in the capacity to write insurance due to other casualty line losses and the 1974 stock market decline, indirectly affected availability; however, these factors would have been insignificant had the predictive ability of the industry been sufficient.

Third, even given the inadequate predictive capability, it is unlikely that the insurance industry's response would have been dramatic increases in premiums or abrupt withdrawal from the market had the base over which to spread the risk been larger. That is, by insurance standards, the number of potential insureds (less than 400,000) is very small. Compared with the number of automobile drivers (over one hundred million), it is miniscule.

Thus, the dilemma faced by the insurance industry in 1974 was this—inability to predict the risk adequately, unavailability of underwriting funds, and a small base across which to spread the risk. Although it would be easy at this point to assume that the blame for the malpractice crisis should fall on the insurers, to do so would beg the question of underlying causes. The American Bar Association's Commission on Medical Professional Liability (ABA/CMPL)* concluded that although the underlying causes were "many and diverse and may never be fully

---

* See Appendix C for a detailed summary of this study.

known," certain other factors could be categorized as either medical or legal.[3]

Medical Causes

Medical factors contributing to the malpractice crisis were: (1) changes in the way medicine was practiced, (2) professional response to the effects of those changes, and (3) the response of patients to the changes. Dramatically sophisticated growth in medical technology and more frequent use of complicated machines and procedures meant that more could be done for the patient or to the patient. While technology resulted in striking gains in medical care, it also increased the risk of more serious adverse results. In addition, the sophistication of medical practice caused an explosion in the number of personnel taking part in patient care, expanding the categories of licensed or credentialed health care providers to at least fifty. Consequently, the involvement of more people in the treatment sequence increased the risk of communication and follow-up errors.

According to the ABA/CMPL, the medical profession responded inadequately to these changes and particularly to the increased risks. Within the medical profession, discipline was either inadequate or non-existent. Once licensed, physicians practiced for life. In most states, incompetence was not grounds for revoking a license; states allowing incompetence as grounds rarely invoked it; and cases based on incompetence often took years to settle. Provided with few alternative mechanisms by which to discipline and having few incentives to do so, licensing boards and medical societies were ineffective in disciplining physicians.

Hospitals responded similarly. Faced with the increasing risk of patient injuries within their walls, hospitals were slow to recognize their responsibilities for medical malpractice. They traditionally made no or inadequate efforts to prevent the occurrence of adverse incidents. Like the licensing boards, they had available no proven mechanisms; like the medical societies, they had few incentives to do so. Only with developing changes in the law and its interpretation have these incentives emerged.

By 1974, patients were responding dramatically to societal changes, including the changes in medical practice. Their fascination with the mechanics of technology reflected their expectations of what medical technology could do. Complex machinery, sophisticated hospitals, and superspecialized personnel should have produced improved health.

When their expectations were not fully met and especially when adverse effects resulted, patients often felt aggrieved. In addition to growing expectations, patients' willingness to learn about health matters increased and thus their knowledge grew. No longer totally mystified by the mechanics of medical care or by its jargon, patients increasingly began to question the quality of their care and to demand that providers of health care services be accountable and responsible for poor outcomes. These demands, in part, reflected: (1) unreasonable expectations regarding the ability of medicine to cure, (2) increased medical specialization and the resultant depersonalization of care, and/or (3) greater litigiousness, i.e., the increased willingness to sue.

Legal Causes

The legal system provided its share of the factors leading to the increasing frequency and severity of claims. Of the factors identified by the ABA/CMPL, one involved the court system and the rules of law, one involved lawyers themselves, and one involved juries. The most important factor, however, was that appellate courts liberalized the substantive and procedural rules of law to give plaintiffs easier access to the courts for establishing entitlement to damages.

The ABA/CMPL noted two significant trends. One dealt with strict liability.

> (1) One who sells any product in a defective condition unreasonably dangerous to the user or consumer or to his property is subject to liability for physical harm thereby caused to the ultimate user or consumer, or to his property, if (a) the seller is engaged in the business of selling such a product, and (b) it is expected to and does reach the user or consumer without substantial change in the condition in which it is sold. (2) The rule stated in Subsection (1) applies although (a) the seller has exercised all possible care in the preparation and sale of his product, and (b) the user or consumer has not bought the product from or entered into any contractual relation with the seller [p. 46].

Prior to 1974, court decisions in product liability cases clearly reflected this trend. The ABA/CMPL presumed that applying the concept of strict liability in tort to medical malpractice would be appropriate, in effect converting the tort liability system to a compensation only system.

The second important trend noted was the increased application of the doctrine of res ipsa loquitur. Literally "the thing speaks for itself," the doctrine means that, in certain instances, the presence of an injury creates the presumption of negligence. For example, patient injury is alleged due to a surgical instrument that is found in the patient and that is identified with the defendant-physician. The application of this rule of law means the injury obviously resulted from negligence. In the not-too-distant past, expert testimony was the sole means by which plaintiffs could show negligence. Failure to produce this expert testimony (i.e., physicians who would testify against other physicians) meant that plaintiffs were precluded from proving their cases. According to the ABA/CMPL, the application of strict liability theories, of res ipsa loquitur, of informed consent, and of other legal rules, including learned treatises, enabled plaintiffs to gain increased access to the courts.

As a result of these legal trends, the medical community identified statutes of limitations and the contingency fee system as factors contributing to the medical malpractice crisis. Statutes of limitations control the amount of time within which a suit must be initiated after an injury. Most states have broadly drawn legislation that is based upon the time an injury is discovered rather than on the time the injury occurred. In addition, many states have statutes governing persons under legal disabilities. For example, a minor could be entitled to bring an action as late as the age of majority plus the otherwise applicable statute of limitations. An individual brain-damaged at birth could theoretically bring a viable action decades later. Consequently, physicians are subject to suit long after injuries occur and long after medical knowledge changes.*

Under the contingency fee system, the insured party and his attorney enter into an agreement whereby the attorney's fees are proportionately related to the recovery; that is, a certain percentage of the recovery is the fee for the attorney. Though vilified by the medical community, the contingency fee system provides those who could not otherwise afford it access to the courts.

Among the factors contributing to the crisis in the mid-1970s, the ABA/CMPL identified the increased number of practicing attorneys

---

* In some states, the statute of limitations may be as short as a year or two with no tolling for minority or disability, and notice of a potential claim may be required even sooner for certain governmental bodies. In some other states, lawsuits may be brought up to the age of majority plus the statute of limitations, with tolling for minority or disability. In still other states, the statute of limitations may not begin running until an injury is discovered or at least until it should reasonably have been discovered. Some jurisdictions extend the statute of limitations when fraud or covering up of acts of negligence is evident. Of course, in theory, the standard of care applied to any particular medical event should be the standard as it existed at the time the care was rendered.

during the preceding decade and the increased number of attorneys experienced in malpractice cases. More than 180,000 new lawyers were admitted to the bar between 1963 and 1974; presently more than 40,000 new attorneys are admitted each year.[4] These numbers indicate an increasing availability of legal services as well as a proportionate increase in those who elect to specialize in medical malpractice. Survival in such an increasingly competitive arena may be a significant consideration. For example, the increase in medical malpractice lawsuits in Massachusetts allegedly occurred concurrently with the passage of that state's automobile no-fault law.[5,6] Attorneys who formerly represented victims in automobile accident or negligence cases apparently began representing victims of alleged medical negligence.

A final legal factor in the malpractice crisis was the increasing tendency of juries to give extremely large damage awards, particularly in cases of severe, permanent injury. Attitudes similar to those of patients—higher expectations of medical technology and the belief that a bad outcome must have been caused by negligent care—may have prevailed in these awards. In addition, juries may have believed that they were redistributing losses to those most able to pay, i.e., to institutions, physicians, and insurers. Whatever the reason, the size of awards exacerbated the insurance dilemma of prediction.

Short-Range Solutions to the Crisis

In direct response to the immediate crisis, health care providers, regulators, and some in the insurance industry developed approaches to assure the continued availability of medical care. As analyzed by the American Bar Association's Fund for Public Education* and reported in January 1977, efforts proceeded in two directions: (1) development of mechanisms to assist the availability of insurance, and (2) development of statutory modifications in tort law.[7] Changes and improvements in these two areas offered continued availability of malpractice insurance.†

Warren and Merritt‡ reported that the most common substantive response to medical malpractice problems was the passage of legislation authorizing joint underwriting associations (JUAs).[8] In 1975 alone,

---

* See Appendix D for a detailed summary of this report.

† See Chapter 3, The Present Situation, for a detailed discussion of the tort reforms enacted.

‡ See Appendix E for a detailed summary of this study.

more than twenty states passed such laws. This underwriting concept forced insurers to provide malpractice coverage and share (pool) any resulting losses subject to recoupment. In exchange, the insurers received greater protection against unrecouped losses and retained the right to carry more lucrative kinds of liability insurance. In most cases, the legislation provided that the JUA be a temporary administrative structure, to be continued only if no better plan emerged. A small number of states, for example, set up state funding instead of, in addition to, or as a backup for the JUA. Such plans avoided potential constitutional problems by requiring insurers to participate in the JUA and by reducing the costs of excess liability coverage.

Other mechanisms with the purpose of assuring insurance availability were also the subject of legislation. Some states authorized reinsurance exchanges that would insure malpractice insurance policies written by member insurers. In return, however, insurers could not terminate or refuse a policy to the extent it could be reinsured. Another plan that was authorized and funded in a few states was the formation of mutual insurance associations owned by physicians. Maryland, for example, created a nonprofit organization, initially funded by a one-time tax of all physicians licensed in the state. The organization's charge included a provision of insurance, the requirement to participate in the JUA, and the ability to require funds from its members to cover losses above premium payment income.

These responses to the crisis had the desired effect—malpractice liability insurance continued to be universally available, although at significantly higher prices, and disruption in medical care did not occur. The system adjusted to higher costs; in general, physicians continued to practice, passing along in increased fees the increased premium costs. However, the unavailability of insurance—the crisis—reflected the changes taking place in the legal and medical care systems and in public expectations of them.

References

1. Department of Health, Education, and Welfare. Medical malpractice: report of the secretary's commission on medical malpractice. Washington, DC: US Government Printing Office, 1973.
2. Curran, WJ. Medical malpractice claims since the crisis of 1975: some good news and some bad. N Engl J Med 309:1107, 1983.
3. American Bar Association. American Bar Association 1977 report of the commission on medical professional liability. Chicago: Author, 1977.

4. American Bar Association (Section of Legal Education and Admissions to the Bar). A review of legal education in the United States, fall, 1982, law schools and bar admission requirements. Chicago: Author, 1983.
5. Chapter 670 of Acts and Resolves of 1970, Massachusetts law.
6. Chapter 90, Section 34-M, Massachusetts General Laws (amended 1972, 1980).
7. American Bar Association's Fund for Public Education. American Bar Association fund for public education report concerning legal topics relating to medical malpractice. Washington, DC: US Department of Health, Education, and Welfare, Public Health Service, 1977.
8. Warren, DG and Merritt, R, eds. A legislator's guide to the medical malpractice issue. Washington, DC: Health Policy Center, Graduate School, Georgetown University, 1976.

Chapter 3

The Present Situation

Charles M. Jacobs and Daniel K. Roberts

Recent proposals advocating the implementation of arbitration and pretrial panels as well as a variety of no-fault plans presume that there is enough wrong with the litigation system to justify establishing an alternative mechanism for resolving medical malpractice claims. Advocates of these approaches view the present system as so flawed that no amount of adjustment can adequately repair it. Although the proponents of alternate mechanisms are still too few to prevail, they will have much more credibility as tort law reforms continue to prove ineffective and as another medical malpractice crisis continues to develop.

The arguments against the present system of litigation stem primarily from two sources, health care professionals and their patients. Health care providers view the system as unpredictable because some injured patients unjustly never receive compensation and because some physicians who are sued are known by their peers to be highly qualified, careful professionals. Medical malpractice judgments seem like a plague that afflicts both the just and the unjust, overcompensating some, undercompensating some, failing to compensate others, and appearing to strike randomly.

Patients also view the litigation system as ineffective, time consuming, and uncertain. To receive compensation for an injury, the patient must recognize the injury, relate the injury to a medical cause, recognize the right to sue in order to show liability, find an attorney willing to take the case, and endure the vicissitudes of the case. If the findings of the California Medical Insurance Feasibility Study (CMIFS),* which randomly sampled medical records for potentially compensable events, were extrapolated to the nation, about one and one-half million compensable events could be predicted annually.[1] The National Association of Insurance Commissioners (NAIC)† reported that the number of claims closed between 1975 and 1978 averaged only slightly over 23,000 annually, thereby illustrating the inefficiency of the present compensation system to identify injuries.[2]

The litigation system as applied to medical malpractice has other deficiencies in addition to its inefficiency as a compensation mechanism. It is, for example, alleged that malpractice suits serve as quality assurance mechanisms—that since the injured patient may sue the provider of care, the provider is more careful than he would have been without the threat of suit. Physicians may consequently order unrelated tests and subject patients to questionably indicated procedures because of the vague threat of suit; however, such defensive practices may cause more harm than benefit in addition to having an adverse effect on costs.

Many elements that brought about the crisis in the mid-1970s continue to exist—factors that are now contributing to the second wave of the medical malpractice crisis. These are:

- The insurance climate is in many respects unchanged from that which produced the crisis in the mid-1970s.
- Society continues to grow increasingly litigious.
- The present litigation system is inefficient as a compensation mechanism and inappropriate as a quality assurance mechanism.
- Attempts to solve the previous crisis concentrated on short-term measures to increase the availability of insurance as well as some fine-tuning of the litigation system, but included no major, comprehensive long-term solutions.
- Limited progress has been made toward alternative mechanisms of conflict resolution in medical malpractice cases.

Representative of the many voices predicting increasing claims, bigger awards, escalating premiums, and greater uncertainty about the availability of insurance was James Ludlam, counsel for the California

---

* See Appendix B for a detailed summary of this study.
† See Appendix A for a detailed discussion of this report.

Hospital Association and a member of the ABA/CMPL.[3] Long before the malpractice situation again attained the status of a full-blown crisis, Ludlam foresaw a new round of problems because of several factors.

> First, the short-term impact of the tort reform measures will wear off. Those measures, never very significant to begin with, have in several cases been held unconstitutional (e.g., limits on total amount of liability, certain changes in the statute of limitations). In addition, inventive attorneys are finding ways to work around them.
>
> Second, as the number of physicians "going bare" is reduced (to perhaps 2% by 1978) and as publicity over the earlier crisis wears off, the incentive to sue and the potential for large judgments appear to be increasing for patients.
>
> Third, increasing consumerism in law is evidenced by an escalation of cases in product liability. Courts are expanding theories under which plaintiffs can sue and recover. This trend toward consumerism is unlikely to be reversed, particularly for medicine.

Finally, Ludlam warned that a new factor in the predicted crisis—provider-owned companies—would be extremely vulnerable because as specialized carriers, they would not have the availability of other lines of insurance against which to spread sudden losses.

In the crisis of the mid-1970s, the scapegoat was generally considered to be the insurance industry, and the response was generally to make insurance available and to make adjustments in tort law. In the present crisis, the finger can no longer be pointed at insurers, especially since many insurers are now provider owned. Tort law reforms are not the solution because of the powerful special interest groups who block, dilute, or strike down any meaningful proposals. As a practical matter, state legislatures will not further alter the balance between patients and providers by again trying to make readjustments in tort law.

Federal Intervention

There was little activity and no enthusiasm for federal intervention in the malpractice crisis of the mid-1970s. As another crisis approaches, some momentum for federal involvement may be building for several reasons. First, the return of the crisis can be taken as evidence that state governments and voluntary mechanisms could not produce meaningful solutions. Second, in the intervening years, there has been a tremendous increase in the federal role in health care. The Professional

Standards Review Organization (PSRO) program and Health Systems Agencies (HSAs) have extended federal involvement in overseeing the delivery, quality, utilization, and organization of health services. Additionally, in an admittedly narrow application, the federal government's acceptance of the liability burden for swine flu vaccines (administered without charge by private physicians or other providers) created a precedent in this area. Thus, as the present crisis escalates, a federal role may be accepted, even if grudgingly so.

Any attempt at federal intervention might be directed either at eliminating the present system of litigation or at making it more efficient. Elimination is the approach taken by no-fault plans that would compensate patients for medically related injuries. This approach eliminates the necessity for finding fault before compensation is awarded. Bills proposing such a no-fault approach were introduced in the United States Congress in 1975 and have been reintroduced with the emergence of another crisis. Most no-fault proposals generally include controls over medical and institutional practices, such as more stringent utilization and quality review or the establishment of institutional risk management programs in order to qualify as federal providers. In return for paying an increasing share of the cost of health care, the federal government will demand to control a portion of that expenditure, as evidenced by Medicare hospital reimbursement regulations apportioning allowable malpractice related reimbursement based on the actual claim history of the Medicare population.

The second form of federal intervention, to make the claims resolution mechanism more efficient, was outlined by Griffin Bell when he was the Attorney General of the United States. The United States Justice Department considered recommending legislation that would have required all states to set up pretrial screening panels to review all malpractice claims before they could be filed. Operating under federally established minimum standards, these panels would have been charged with weeding out nonmeritorious claims and expediting payment for meritorious claims. Resolution of claims in court could still have been pursued, but substantial penalties would have been imposed on those who continued and then lost cases that had received an adverse panel decision.

Data compiled by the American Medical Association indicated that twenty-five states had established screening panels of some type by 1977, although most were voluntary. Challenges based on the constitutionality of these panels, however, have been successful in Florida, Illinois, Utah, Missouri, Ohio, and Pennsylvania.

Risk Management*

Recent efforts to deal with increasing liability costs by organizing risk management or loss control programs have come from professional and hospital associations, from insurance companies, and from state legislatures. In 1980, the American Hospital Association estimated that 51.5 percent of the nation's hospitals had formal organized risk management programs.

State legislatures have moved hesitantly into the area of institutional risk management. In 1976, Florida became the first of only a handful of states to require hospitals to have an internal risk management system. Specifically, Florida required a system of mandatory reporting of adverse medical incidents to a duly qualified risk manager. Each hospital was also required to create a medical incident committee to rule on compensable events and the degree of liability involved.

In addition, when faced with increased premiums or difficulty in purchasing malpractice insurance, many health care providers such as hospitals, hospital associations, professional societies, and shared service groups are making the decision to self-insure. Conventional insurance, however, is often purchased as an umbrella above the primary assumption of some limited amount of risk. The key required for the success of such a program is the strong support of all participants—hospital administrators, boards of directors, and medical staff members.

Although no thorough evaluations of these efforts have been done, risk management makes good sense. It offers a means for decreasing professional and/or institutional costs and for improving the quality of patient care. Risk management is, therefore, in the best interests of health care providers, the insurance industry, and ultimately patients.

References

1. Mills, DH, ed. Report on the medical insurance feasibility study. San Francisco: California Medical Association, 1977.
2. Sowka, MP, ed. Malpractice claims: final compilation: medical malpractice closed claims, 1975–1978. Brookfield, WI: National Association of Insurance Commissioners, 1980.
3. American Bar Association. American Bar Association 1977 report of the commission on medical professional liability. Chicago: Author, 1977.

---

* See Section 3, Managing the Risk, for detailed discussions of this topic.

Understanding the Law

To say the least, medical practitioners are uncomfortable when they must participate in the legal arena either as a defendant or as an expert witness. We describe the history of medical liability, define the rules that govern the litigation process, and delineate the responsibilities of the various participants. Understanding the law and familiarity with its process, procedures, and rules will give physicians a grasp of the system that has such far-reaching consequences for the practice of medicine.

Chapter 4

The Historic Basis
of Medical-Legal Liability*

Edgar A. Reed

Several years ago, Malcolm C. Todd, a past president of the American Medical Association (AMA), stated, "The cost of medical malpractice insurance is the biggest problem facing the young physician entering practice today."[1] That statement, as true now as it was then, is a tragic commentary when a physician's biggest problem must be stated in terms of a potential financial loss rather than the quality of health care being delivered to patients. A significant cause of this dilemma is due, in part, to most physicians' head-in-the-sand attitude with regard to how the law impacts on them and their profession.

If you were to enter the law office of any successful plaintiff's attorney who is trying a significant number of medical malpractice cases, not only would you find a medical library almost any physician could be proud of, but a brief conversation with this lawyer would reveal an extensive, sophisticated knowledge of medicine and medical terminology. Fortunately for physicians, an increasing number of defense attorneys are also learning more about medicine. The point is that an ever increasing number of lawyers are learning more about medicine because it is especially advantageous for them to do so.

But how many doctors even have a single monograph in their library dealing with how the law affects their professional activities—how it

---

* An earlier version appeared in the Journal of Legal Medicine 6(10):50, 1977.

affects their very livelihood. Now I am neither suggesting nor advocating that physicians should hurry out and enroll in law school, for that kind of logic might suggest that everyone who drives a car should also be an automotive engineer. But it is an anachronism, it seems to me, that so many physicians, who seriously study the stock market or real estate as they pursue their various financial ventures, know little or nothing about how the law affects their professional activities. This discussion is directed at providing an introduction to some of those elements of the law that are causing so much concern.

Early Common Law

With only a few exceptions, the basis of medical-legal liability is found in what is referred to as the law of torts. However, not even this century's leading law professor on that subject found it easy to define either *tort law* or a *tort,* and it would be presumptuous to say any more than Professor William Prosser's classic textbook on the subject: "a tort is a civil wrong, other than breach of contract, for which the court will provide a remedy in the form of an action for damages" (p. 2).[2] Regardless of what modified definition is used, tort law cannot be well understood without some knowledge and appreciation of the history of the common law.

Long before the development of the common law, earliest tribal or communal law depended solely on local practice and custom for controlling members' actions.[3] Later, people's rights, duties, and penalties for failure to perform as required were regulated by codes of conduct. Probably one of the oldest known codes is the Code of Hammurabi. Developed by that Babylonian king some twenty centuries before the Christian era, the code required that a doctor's hands be cut off if he treated a man with a metal knife and the patient died.[4] Even the ancient Mosaic Code of the Israelites, which is barely eight centuries younger, perpetuated further the concept of lex talionis or the law of the talon by demanding "an eye for an eye and a tooth for a tooth."[5-7]

The development of the form and principles of law we use today in America can probably be traced from no farther back than the 1200s, or nearly two centuries after the Norman conquest of the British Isles in 1066. The next several hundred years saw the development of the court system of modern-day England from the Common Pleas Courts to the Royal Courts (or Bench). During this developmental period, these courts established a variety of procedural rules. Those who considered themselves wronged were permitted access to the court only after they had complied with these very formal and rigidly stylized procedures. Among these procedures was the requirement that the offense charged should be in the form of a specific *writ* before the plaintiff could be heard by the court. To summon a defendant into court, the plaintiff was forced to choose one of the prescribed writs then available and attempt to apply it to the particular facts of his case. Frequently, there existed no appropriate writ (or pigeonhole); consequently, the complaining party was denied a hearing and an access to justice or was forced to be considerably innovative or to create *legal fictions* before the court would administer its type of justice.

However, more important than the development of the *system* of courts with their rules of procedure was the accumulation of a vast body of decisions in both criminal and civil cases dating back to about 1300 during the reign of Edward I. Published during this period was the first *Year Book* which consisted simply of a compilation of informal notes of cases and comments made by lawyers and students. This body of decisions and the custom of *applying* these prior decisions of the royal courts to new cases became known as the *common law* and was later brought to this country by the early colonists from England.

The law of torts is an outgrowth of the ancient law of the British Isles when there was no differentiation between a crime and a civil wrong. Historically, all wrongs were crimes against the crown and were classified as either felonies or crimes of trespass. From this latter category of trespass, which was modified by ecclesiastical law (or equity), tort law has gradually evolved.

Trespass and *Case*

The two writs considered the forerunners of present-day torts were known as *action of trespass* and *action of trespass on the case,* or, more simply, *trespass* and *case.*[2] Trespass was initially a crime of the nature of a misdemeanor and allowed the king's court to try and to punish those guilty of serious and forcible breaches of the king's peace. From this action resulted the first money damages being awarded to the injured party. So it was that any man who threw rocks at his neighbor's house and broke the windows would not only be tried for his direct intentional injury to his neighbor's property as a breach of the king's peace (a criminal action), but he would also be required by the court to make the house as whole as it was before or to pay for its repair (a civil action for the tort).

But the writ of trespass could not apply to all the injuries those rocks caused. What of the consequences if some of those same rocks rolled off the roof onto the street below where they remained for days? Later, those rocks might cause a horse to stumble and throw his rider, resulting in the rider breaking his leg. The rock thrower had no intention of injuring the horseman, nor were the thrown rocks directed at either the horse or his rider. Finally, the injury the rider suffered was not an immediate effect of the rock throwing but rather was remote from the act by several days. For all these reasons, the elements of trespass could not apply; therefore, there was no legal relief for the injured rider who suffered pain, paid his own medical bills, and lost money from his business. Hence, in an effort to provide an appropriate remedy for those injuries sustained when the wrongful act was neither direct nor immediate, the writ of trespass on the case was developed which then permitted this hapless fellow to haul the rock thrower into court.

From this early beginning over six hundred years ago has evolved present-day tort law. The object of tort law has always been the determination of the legally protected rights of the individual person, his property, and his reputation which must not be interfered with or invaded. Therefore, within the basic precepts of tort law are the components of medical-legal liability, the most important of these being (1) intentional interference, (2) negligence, and (3) strict liability.

Intentional Interference

The tort of intentional interference (sometimes more simply referred to as an *intentional tort*) is a direct outgrowth of the ancient writ of trespass. In its evolution, however, the original crime of trespass, where the injury was direct, has been modified to emphasize the *intent* of the wrongdoer in contrast to the lack of intent to do harm in the tort of negligence. A variety of terms originally associated with trespass have been continued into the modern classification of intentional torts, e.g., assault, battery, false imprisonment, defamation, deceit, and fraud.

In general, the law deals much more harshly with those accused of an intentional tort than other torts. In many cases of intentional tort, it is unnecessary for the plaintiff to prove an injury resulted from the tortious act in order to obtain a judgment for damages. That the act was performed with an *intent* to do harm is considered to be both legally and morally wrong. Although the burden of proving the defendant's *intent* is often one of the plaintiff's greatest obstacles, it is frequently sufficient to show only that the act was a practical joke which misfired or that the act was directed toward someone else but it nevertheless caused an injury to the plaintiff. The distinction is that the defendant intended to perform the act, as opposed to his negligent performance of the act, which is sometimes referred to as *transferring the intent*.

Another important distinction between an intentional tort and negligence is that negligence involves a departure from usual and customary standards of behavior. In a negligence case, expert witnesses will establish whether or not such a departure occurred, which is not required in a case alleging an intentional tort. For a surgeon to remove an organ during surgery without the specific permission of the patient constitutes the intentional tort of battery. The plaintiff-patient is not required to introduce testimony by an expert witness that removal of the organ did not conform to usual and customary standards.

The intentional tort of deceit is quite often referred to today as either fraud or misrepresentation.* To show deceit requires the following:

1. the defendant knowingly made a false representation;
2. the false representation was made in order to benefit the person making the representation or to cause harm to another person;
3. the plaintiff relied on the misrepresentation as true; and
4. the plaintiff was injured as a result of his reliance.

Two examples should be adequate to illustrate how this intentional tort might be applied to the practice of medicine.

1. A physician finds he left a foreign body in a patient during an earlier procedure but fails to tell the patient the real cause of his symptoms while obtaining consent for the second surgical procedure.
2. A physician fails to disclose the diagnosis of a malignancy to a patient who then, in reliance on a benign diagnosis, conducts his affairs in a way that results in an injury to himself and/or his estate.

In neither case is the testimony of an expert witness required. Perhaps even more important, however, most professional liability insurance carriers will not provide a physician with defense counsel or reimbursement for damages when the cause of action is an intentional tort.

---

* Although many authors hasten to point out fine distinctions between these two, their common features are sufficient to treat them collectively in this discussion.

Finally, a brief mention without a detailed discussion should be made of the recent trend of plaintiffs to seek not only enforcement of their civil rights but also damages where these civil rights have been denied them. The possibility of being a defendant in an action where the plaintiff alleges one or more of his constitutional rights have been denied is an ever increasing threat. Additional emphasis has been given to these and other civil rights by the Civil Rights Act(s) of 1964 and 1965, which even provide for criminal penalties as well as civil remedies for infringing on certain rights of persons.[8,9]

Negligence

Negligence as a separate and distinct tort is a relative child to the law, for not until around 1825 was the concept applied in this country, primarily against the railroads as they began to take their toll of the lives of sheep, cows, and men.[10] This evolution seemed both natural and necessary, for the older actions of trespass and case could no longer be applied to the issues confronting the courts, even with the attempted distinction between intentional and unintended torts. The category of unintended tort ultimately gave way to negligence as the descendant of case action, while the classification of intentional tort remains as a vestige of trespass action.

But how does the law define negligence so as to permit its application as a separate and independent basis of tort liability? Negligence may be considered as "conduct which involves an unreasonably great risk of causing damage" (p. 42),[11] or perhaps better, "conduct which falls below the standard established by law for the protection of others against unreasonable risk of harm."[12] Medical negligence then can be defined as medical care that falls below the established standard of care expected of similarly trained physicians for the protection of similar patients under like circumstances.

Before the negligent conduct of a wrongdoer can be applied in a cause of civil litigation, however, more is required than merely citing a definition and complaining of negligence. There are, in fact, four distinct elements necessary to show negligence as a cause of action. These are:

1. that the actor owes a duty, or standard of conduct, to the injured party to protect the injured from unreasonable risk;
2. that the actor failed to conform to that duty or standard of conduct;

3. that the negligent act was the *proximate cause* of the injury to the complaining party; and
4. that the complaining party suffered actual loss or injury which can be measured as money damages.[2]

Through common usage during the past several decades, medical negligence, or that medical conduct below the established standard of care, has been euphemized as *mal* or bad. Hence, the term *malpractice* has become the popular term for the more correct one of *medical negligence.*

The first recorded action brought for medical negligence in England occurred in 1374, while the first American case occurred in 1794 in Connecticut.[13,14] Although there were several American cases during the late eighteenth century and early nineteenth century in which former patients sought to recover damages for their injuries alleged to be the proximate result of medical negligence, the most frequently quoted early case dealing with medical negligence is probably *Pike v. Honsinger,* which occurred in 1898.[15] In that case, the Court of Appeals of New York stated four distinct principles of law that continue to impact, with some modification, on the daily practice of medicine more than eight decades later and have provided a standard against which many similar cases have been tried. At the time of trial, Mr. Pike sought damages from Dr. Honsinger for the negligent treatment of his injured knee. The New York Court of Appeals in reversing the decision of the lower court and ordering a new trial said:

> [1] A physician . . . by taking charge of a case, impliedly represents that he possesses . . . that reasonable degree of learning and skill . . . ordinarily possessed by physicians in the locality . . . and which is ordinarily . . . necessary to qualify him . . . in . . . practicing medicine . . . . It becomes his duty to use reasonable care and diligence in the exercise of his skill and his learning . . . . [2] he is under the . . . obligation to use his best judgement exercising his skill and applying his knowledge . . . . [3] he is bound to keep abreast of the times, and . . . departure from approved methods in general use, if it injures the patient, will render him liable . . . . [4] the giving of proper instructions to his patient in relation to conduct, exercise, and the use of an injured limb [p. 762].

Strict Liability

The concept of strict liability is probably the purest survivor of the early writ of trespass on the case. Early tort law was much more concerned with providing an appropriate remedy and keeping peace among the citizens than with determining responsibility or fault. In fact it might be said that today's no-fault compensation is a direct vestige of English common law case. A clear expression of this concept was made by a late seventeenth century English court which said, "In all civil acts, the law doth not so much regard the intent of the actor, as the loss and damage of the party suffering" (p. 221).[16]

During the subsequent two hundred years, the law inexorably moved toward the identification and recognition of fault to form the basis of legal liability for damages. Although the theory of negligence was developing rapidly, there remained many who continued to argue that a finding of liability without fault provided a more equitable basis for assessing damages than requiring a determination of fault. Even today legal scholars continue this debate, and there are some indications that negligence is rapidly losing to strict liability (no fault) as the easier and more equitable basis for determining damages.[17–20]

However, during the past century the tendency has been to discard the doctrine of "never any liability without fault." In its place is a growing social policy that seeks to impose liability on the party who can best bear the loss even though there is no fault. This trend can be considered a natural outgrowth of holding strictly liable those who engage in dangerous activity (e.g., blasting), those who keep animals (e.g., zoos and guard dogs), and those who operate dangerous equipment (e.g., heavy construction). The basic liability in all these examples is that they create an undue risk of harm to other members of the community.

To my knowledge, the substantive legal doctrine of strict liability has not been directly applied by an American court in an action brought by a plaintiff-patient against a defendant-physician. Nevertheless, this doctrine is affecting how the courts determine liability. For example, the product liability doctrine which affects the pharmaceutical and medical appliance industries is a hybrid of strict liability and warranty. Even more important, however, is that the doctrine of strict liability is influencing many courts and arbitration bodies to look to the party who can best afford the loss which the patient has suffered. Indeed many pretrial settlements appear to be paying for damages even when there is no evidence of negligence.

Conclusion

A greater appreciation of how the law of torts has developed over the years gives a basis for understanding how it impacts on the practice of medicine today. Certainly the law is living and ever changing; and while we may disagree or be dissatisfied with the law, it does respond eventually to the pressures of society through what is euphemistically called public policy. In Western society, persons who are injured will always demand some compensation, especially when the injured party is innocent of any fault. In the future, the forum in which deliberations take place, the procedural steps taken, and the criteria applied may only remotely resemble the present-day medical malpractice trial. Nevertheless, physicians must be aware of and be actively involved in shaping the public policy and resulting law that impact on their profession.

The future will bring new decisions and statutes on death and the terminally ill patient.[21-23] The final chapter on abortion has not yet been written. The procedural rule of res ipsa loquitur and the negligence theory of informed consent have developed and been applied to medicine.[24-26] The corporate responsibility of hospitals for the actions of staff physicians has been affirmed.[27] There will be much more!

We in medicine can never afford to lack compassion for our fellow man, but neither can we afford to be complacent or ignorant of the law as it affects our life's work. If we are, we will surely figuratively suffer the fate of our ancestors under King Hammurabi and lose many good *hands* from the ranks of our noble profession.

References

1. Todd, MC. Keynote address before Association of Military Surgeons of the US. Washington, DC, November 1, 1976.
2. Prosser, WL. Handbook of the law of torts, ed 4. St Paul, MN: West Publishing Co, 1971.
3. Kempin, FG, Jr. Historical introduction to Anglo-American law, ed 2. St Paul, MN: West Publishing Co, 1973.
4. Webel, S. The world's earliest "journal of legal medicine." J Leg Med 3(2):36, 1975.
5. Exodus. 21:23–25.
6. Deuteronomy. 19:21.
7. Leviticus. 24:19–22.
8. 78 Stat. 241.
9. 79 Stat. 437.
10. Winfield, PH. The history of negligence in the law of torts. Law Q Rev 42:184, 1926.
11. Terry, HT. Negligence. Harv Law Rev 29:40, 1915.
12. Second Restatement of Torts Section 282, 1964.
13. Stetler, CJ. The history of reported medical professional liability cases. Temple Law Q 30(4):366, 1957.

14. *Cross v. Guthrey,* 2 Root 90, 1774.
15. *Pike v. Honsinger,* 49 NE 760, 155 NY 201, 1898.
16. *Lamber v. Bessey,* 83 Eng Rep's 220, 1681.
17. Lyons, LJ. No fault for all general liability lines is studied. National Underwriter, November 15, 1974.
18. O'Connell, J. Expanding no-fault beyond auto insurance. Va Law Rev 59:747, 1973.
19. Havighurst, CC and Tancredi, LR. Medical adversity insurance—a no-fault approach to medical malpractice and quality assurance. Milbank Memorial Fund Q 51:125, 1973.
20. Sacoccia, P. No-fault malpractice insurance. N Engl J Med 289(20):1096, 1973.
21. *In the Matter of Karen Quinlan,* 355 A2d 647, NJ, 1976.
22. *Superintendent of Belchertown State School v. Saikewicz,* 370 NE2d 417, Mass, 1977.
23. *In re Dinnerstein,* 380 NE2d 134, Mass, 1978.
24. Black, HC. Black's law dictionary, ed 4. St Paul, MN: West Publishing Co, 1975.
25. *Canterbury v. Spence,* 464 F2d 772, DC, certiorari denied, 409 US 1064, 1972.
26. *Cobbs v. Grant,* 502 P2d 1, 8 Cal 3d 229, 1972.
27. *Darling v. Charleston Community Memorial Hospital,* 211 NE2d 253, Ill, 1975.

Chapter 5

Anatomy of a Lawsuit

Jeffrey A. Shane

Physicians often respond inappropriately when a malpractice claim or lawsuit is threatened or actually filed. I believe these responses are grounded in physicians' almost irrational fear of the legal system because it is a powerful but unknown entity; they do not understand either the underlying process or the guiding rules of the legal system. There are a variety of comparisons that may prove instructive: analyzing the law like a game with rules to be learned; viewing the law like a stage play with roles to be studied; examining the law like a specimen with parts to be dissected. My goal is not to teach physicians to be lawyers; rather, I want to render the law a less imposing structure by using an analogy familiar to physicians. In presenting the basic anatomy of a lawsuit, I shall point out the gross characteristics as well as introduce some of the terminology and finer points.

Lawsuits begin months or years before they formally end in litigation. The practitioner gets early indications from the patient who is extremely dissatisfied with her care, from the letter that is written to the physician or to one of the medical societies, or from the attorney who requests medical records. While these clues are technically not part of the lawsuit itself, they can significantly affect a subsequent lawsuit, especially if statements are made or admissions given. In addition, insurance policies may require the physician to notify the carrier when he is aware of a potential claim. To protect his insurance coverage and to make his case defensible, the physician must know what his responsibilities are under his malpractice insurance policy when he becomes aware of an adverse outcome that may be the subject of a lawsuit. Early investigation of the surrounding event may make the case substantially more defensible should a lawsuit be filed.

Some states and jurisdictions require that a case first be presented to a prelitigation screening panel or for arbitration. The claimant must present her case to these legislatively established bodies. Almost always there is a provision that in the event the outcome is unsatisfactory, resort to court is available.

Complaint, Summons, Answer

In most jurisdictions, the lawsuit technically begins when the plaintiff files a formal complaint. The complaint must be filed with the appropriate court and must list the allegations, facts, and legal points

> upon which the plaintiff bases his right to legal relief against the person or persons named as defendants. The complaint may include such things as: an outline of the events that occurred in chronological order; a succinct description of the defendant's actions (or lack of actions) allegedly constituting negligence or malpractice; and an allegation of damages and injuries sustained by the plaintiff as a result of the defendant's conduct [p. 25].[1]

Once the complaint is filed, the court issues a summons, a demand for an answer to the points and issues raised by the plaintiff. The defendant is served with (officially receives) the summons from a process server or law enforcement official. This document must not be taken lightly. It deserves the immediate attention of the involved health care provider. The summons often specifies a time limit for responding, and there are rather stringent penalties for failure to do so.

The physician should immediately consult an attorney who can appropriately answer such a legal document. This attorney may be chosen either by the physician or by the insurance carrier. Such action is extremely important in order not to prejudice the case or to cause a judgment against the health care provider by default. Legal consultation is appropriate regardless of how frivolous the claim might seem to the physician since judgments by default, generally speaking, do not take into consideration the actual merits of the claim.

In answering the complaint, the defendant and his attorney prepare a written response that

> denies or admits each of the allegations contained in the complaint. In addition, the answer may contain allegations of facts or circumstances not

referred to in the complaint, which may serve to exonerate the defendant or to bar the plaintiff from recovery . . . . The plaintiff's allegations may be denied or admitted in whole or in part; to the extent that the defendant admits allegations, these matters need not be proved by the plaintiff at trial [p. 25].

Should the defendant fail to deny an allegation or dispute a fact set forth in the complaint, this omission may be considered as an admission of that point.

Discovery

Answering the summons with specific reference to the allegations in the complaint begins the process of discovery. The purpose of this phase of the lawsuit is to lay open for a full disclosure all of the facts and events surrounding the allegations in the complaint.* There are a number of appropriate procedural devices that may be used by both plaintiff and defense counsel to discover the elements of their adversary's case: document production, oral depositions, interrogatories, requests for admission, physical and mental examinations.†

The plaintiff's attorney has the right to request that any medical records or other relevant health care documents be produced. If the plaintiff's attorney has done a careful job in preparing for the case, he already has the relevant medical records and has had them reviewed by someone competent to render an opinion about the merits of the case. Likewise, defense counsel has the right to request the documents that are the basis of the plaintiff's case.

Should the requested documents not be produced, the court may issue a subpoena requiring the individual to appear personally and to bring with him any pertinent documents in his possession that are not protected or privileged. Which documents are, in fact, protected from inspection by the opposing side varies from jurisdiction to jurisdiction. So that the case is not inappropriately prejudiced, the involved person should consult counsel about whether the documents in his possession are or are not protected.

Defense counsel has the right to obtain information from the plaintiff and any other witnesses she will use to support her case. Likewise, the

---

* Since exact procedures vary substantially from jurisdiction to jurisdiction, the physician should, early in the case, discuss all the aspects of his own jurisdiction with his counsel.

† See Chapter 6, Participating in the Legal Process: A Guide for the Defendant-Physician, for a detailed discussion.

plaintiff's attorney has the right to talk to all personnel who were involved in the care of the patient during the relevant time periods, as well as any other witnesses the defense will use to support their case. Both sides may question these individuals by taking formal, oral depositions. An oral deposition is essentially sworn testimony, admissible in court, that the involved person gives before an individual qualified to record this information (court reporter).* Counsel for both sides are present at these proceedings. The use of the deposition will be dictated by the rules of the court.

In some jurisdictions, expert witnesses may be asked hypothetical questions that are obviously based upon the facts as perceived by the questioning attorney. The defendant-physician can greatly help his attorney prepare to depose a witness, and ultimately to defend the case, by laying out clearly all of the relevant facts and by educating him about the medical aspects of the case. The attorney must be fully briefed so that he can formulate appropriate hypothetical questions as well as be fully prepared for any contingency that may arise during these proceedings.

The television style trial-by-surprise is generally eliminated long before the case goes to an actual courtroom. Virtually all of the information and opinions to be brought out are available, and a substantial portion is in the court record. However, the attorneys for one side or the other are not necessarily going to ask every question at the deposition that they are planning or considering asking at the trial. Rather, the discovery deposition affords counsel for both sides the opportunity to ask about the facts and opinions that they feel may be relevant and for the other side to cross-examine the witness at that time.

Additional information may be obtained during the discovery period from interrogatories, mental and physical examinations, and requests for admission. Interrogatories, similar to depositions in their purpose, are written questions that require written answers from parties on the other side. Physicians must work with their attorneys not only in preparing interrogatories for the plaintiff and her witnesses but also in answering queries from the opposition. A mental or physical examination of the injured plaintiff may be requested by the defendant and ordered by the court if there is some question about the extent, per-

---

* Before attending any such deposition or other proceeding in the case, the health care provider and other personnel should be certain to consult with their legal counsel to be advised about properly preparing for their testimony and about protecting their rights.

manence, or even the existence of the plaintiff's alleged injuries. Requests for admission ask the opposing party to agree in advance that certain facts are undisputed and that certain documents are genuine.

During the course of this discovery process, one or more court hearings may be requested by one side or the other for clarification of certain legal matters or may be required by the court to be advised of the progress of the proceedings and to rule on specific questions of law. When specific points of law are in question, the court usually requires both sides to prepare legal briefs explaining and justifying their position on the particular legal matter. Unless the court has been petitioned to protect from public knowledge certain aspects of the case by, for example, a protective order, the information obtained during discovery proceedings may become public record filed in the court documents.

Ideally, the court maintains fairly tight control of the proceedings and sets forth specific dates by which it expects discovery to be completed. While these schedules often cause some inconvenience to the involved parties, they help avoid unnecessary delays. When the discovery process is finally closed, the court does not allow it to be reopened without showing good cause, i.e., matters coming to light that were not previously known or possible to be known by one side or the other. So that the court can appropriately schedule the trial and estimate how much time will be required to complete it, the parties may be required to reconvene at the court for a pretrial hearing to present briefly to the court the relevant data obtained during discovery.

Settlement

From the time of the initial complaint, suggestions for settling the case may be made by either side. Many factors influence the decision of whether or not to settle a case, including, but not limited to:

- the merits of the case;
- the jurisdiction in which it is to be tried;
- the amount of damages the plaintiff has sustained;
- the amount of settlement that can be reached;
- the limits of the liability policy; and
- personality factors, such as how good a witness an individual will be and how much sympathy might be evoked by the facts in the case.

The health care provider should inspect his insurance policy to determine whether he has any choice in the decision about settlement of the case. To be assured that his rights are being fully protected, the physician may opt to have his own counsel in addition to the counsel appointed by the insurance carrier. This decision is based on such factors as the physician's confidence in his appointed counsel, the limits of his insurance policy, the amount of damages demanded, and the predicted outcome of the trial, which is based on what has come out during discovery. While the defense and costs are covered by the insurer, separately employed counsel is generally not covered by insurance policies and must be paid for by the physician himself.

Settlement, therefore, is not just a tactical problem. Both plaintiff and defendant have substantial costs in continuing the case and proceeding to trial.

Trial

Following these formalities, a trial date is set, and assuming all things go smoothly, the trial will begin. Most malpractice trials are jury trials, although there are exceptions (e.g., lawsuits against the federal government under the Federal Tort Claims Act). The parties usually may opt out of a jury trial if both sides so desire. The jury determines the facts while the judge interprets the law. If there is no jury requested or if, by statute, the case is tried before the judge alone then he performs both functions. If the trial is by jury, then selection of the jury begins. Potential jurors are questioned by the attorneys or the judge, a process known as voir dire, literally "to speak the truth." Although the actual process is highly technical, it is basically an attempt to find a specified number of impartial members of the community to determine which side presents a more believable case.

Once those who will render a verdict on the disputed points of fact and law are determined, both plaintiff and defense counsel present opening statements.

> The opening statement is designed to describe to the jury an outline of what each side of the case intends to present in support of its claim. The purposes include: alerting the jury to the legal character of the case, describing the issues of fact and evidentiary items that will be offered to prove the existence of those facts, and arousing general interest among the jurors in the case itself . . . . Opening statements are limited to a recital of facts that are intended to be proven by that party, and it is not permissible to argue issues of law or to instruct the manner in which disputed issues of fact should be resolved [p. 28].[1]

After opening statements, the plaintiff through her counsel will present her case, often referred to as the *case in chief.* By the testimony of witnesses called, both factual and expert, and by the presentation of physical, demonstrative, and circumstantial evidence, the plaintiff attempts to establish all of the components of her claim. Briefly,

> evidence is anything that serves to make facts clear to human understanding . . . . The major requisite for admissibility of evidence at trial is that the fact or evidence offered be relevant to an issue in the trial. Evidence is deemed relevant if it is 'probative'; that is, if the offered evidence would render some fact more probable after its introduction . . . . there are instances in which such evidence is not allowed. First, some evidence is not permitted because it unduly arouses the jury's prejudice or sympathy . . . . Second, an attorney's line of inquiry may create a side issue that distracts the jury's attention from the principal issues at hand . . . . Third, some matters which an attorney may want to submit at trial are not allowed because of the court's concern for time and economy [pp. 34–35].[1]

Defense counsel may cross-examine each witness who presents evidence at the time of his testimony, and specific points may be narrowed down by redirect questioning and recross-examination. The judge rules on points of law, on the propriety of the proceedings, and on procedural aspects which one or the other side may feel have been violated.

At several points during the trial, either may make certain requests of the court in the form of motions for directed verdict, mistrial, etc. For example, at the close of the plaintiff's case, the defense may make one of several motions, alleging that the plaintiff has failed to make a case.

> The plaintiff must present a prima facie case; that is, assuming the truth of the evidence presented, the case must be enough to suppport a verdict against the defendant and recovery of damages [p. 29].[1]

These motions are often procedural, seldom successful, but important to the overall management of the case. The physician should be aware of why these various legal tactics are undertaken. However, he should make a note of his queries, for it would be inappropriate to interrupt counsel while he is directly attending to the events of the trial.

After the plaintiff presents her case and the judge rules on related motions, the defense presents its case. The defense explains its side of the case using the same tools as the plaintiff: the direct examination, cross-examination, redirect examination of both factual and expert witnesses, and the presentation of physical, demonstrative, and circumstantial evidence.

Following the defendant's case in chief, additional rebuttal testimony may be presented by either or both sides, and additional motions may be made by either side. When all testimony has been heard, plaintiff and defense counsel then make closing arguments, recapping all the testimony the jury has heard and summarizing for the jury their particular side of the case. The judge then instructs the jurors about the relevant legal principles that they are to follow in reaching their verdict. The jury then retires (goes to another, private room) and deliberates (attempts to reach a decision about the merits of the case). Once the jurors have reached a verdict, they present it to the court. In most jurisdictions, unless the judge finds their verdict to be so unreasonable that he is required to rule otherwise, the verdict is entered by the clerk.

Appeal, Countersuit

Either or both sides may immediately or within specified periods of time make various motions to the court including the request for a new trial and appeal of the verdict. The entire verdict may be appealed or a portion of it, e.g., the amount of money damages.

> Assuming that the motion for a new trial is denied, the attorney representing the losing side may make application to the appropriate appellate court for review of the court decision. The appeal may be based upon a number of allegations, but the two most commonly asserted are that the trial court improperly charged the jury as to the applicable law, or that the verdict is contrary to the weight of the evidence presented in the case .... Only a minority of malpractice decisions are overturned on appeal .... The appellate court does not normally interfere with a finding of fact by the jury .... In most cases, a reversal of a trial court decision results in a remanding of the case back to trial court for litigation a second time [pp. 30–31].[1]

Tactical decisions based on the likelihood of success on appeal, the potential costs of such an appeal, and other social and legal ramifications of the verdict as rendered should be discussed with counsel.

Some physicians, after winning a jury trial or after the court dismisses a case, have brought countersuits against the plaintiffs or their attorneys or both.

> Physician-defendant countersuits may be brought on a number of legal theories, including defamation (the physician claims the patient's wrongful suit injured the physician's reputation or character); malicious prosecution (the patient allegedly filed suit only to torment the physician and without any reasonable basis in fact to support the claim); and abuse of process (the patient or patient's attorney is alleged to have used the courts for a wrongful purpose) [p. 181].[2]

Until recently, physicians' countersuits were largely unsuccessful, because the law did not want to create any obstacles that might "inhibit patients with legitimate grievances from seeking redress in the courts" (p. 33).[3] Although since 1976 the law has appeared to be undergoing revision by moving toward affirming the physician's "right not to be sued without reasonable cause" (p. 132), most cases continue to be unsuccessful.[1]

Adversary System

Probably the hardest aspect of the legal system for the physician to understand is the adversarial atmosphere in which the law operates. The key is to realize that the law functions to make the gray areas of human interaction black and white, to determine who has presented the strongest, most believable case and not to pursue absolute truth.

> As physicians are taught the scientific method of examination, assessment, conclusion, and action, attorneys learn to question everything. Nothing is absolute until shown and established in court, and even then it is subject to appeal [p. 3].[1]

To carry this idea further,

> To the medical practitioner, a disputed matter is resolved by a concentrated search for 'the truth,' utilizing accepted scientific method. A similar dispute in a legal context, on the other hand, is not necessarily resolved in terms of a cooperative quest for 'the truth' or 'the answer.' Rather, the American legal system is premised on the assumption that opposing points of view will be ably presented by attorneys who advocate the strongest case for the client and, concomitantly, challenge the opposing litigant's case. While sometimes 'truth' and the final judgment in a lawsuit are synonymous, the search for abstract truth is not the attorney's primary mission [p. 33].[1]

References

1. James, AE, ed. Legal medicine with special reference to diagnostic imaging. Baltimore: Urban and Schwarzenberg, 1980.
2. Fineberg, KS, Peters, JD, Willson, JR, et al. Obstetrics/gynecology and the law. Ann Arbor: Health Administration Press, 1984.
3. Taub, S. Doctors are suing lawyers and some are winning. CT Med 47(1):33, 1983.

Chapter 6

Actors in the Medical-Legal Drama[*]

· Margaret L. Roberts

The physician who finds himself the defendant in a malpractice action often views the surrealistic events surrounding the experience as a drama. Although such an analogy has certain drawbacks, the parallels between a dramatic production and a legal one are numerous enough to warrant using it to explore the human element of a lawsuit—namely, the people, their roles, motivations, and interactions.

Defendant

The defendant-doctor is abruptly, unexpectedly cast into one of the starring roles of the legal drama, one for which he did not choose to audition. He enters the production with a great deal of emotion. His professional integrity is being challenged in a public forum. He experiences enormous frustration, hostility, and, although he would not like to admit it, overwhelming fear. He perceives the plaintiff to be ignorant and ungrateful and the plaintiff's attorney to be the enemy—arrogant and with ethics, intelligence, and medical knowledge all at the same depth.

* The author would like to acknowledge the significant contribution of Marden G. Dixon's "Rules for Redistribution of the Wealth: The Physician's Responsibility in Medical-Legal Matters," which was presented at the twenty-ninth annual ACOG meeting, held in Las Vegas, Nevada, April 25–30, 1981.

Few physicians can carry the image of a Dr. Kildare, Marcus Welby, or Trapper John over into a foreign setting. Although they exude complete confidence and competence when performing in their own arena, surrounded by patients and peers, they can quickly lose that image when forced to recite their lines from the pragmatic legal platform.

Defendant-physicians are not innocent pawns in the legal drama for they play an important role in perpetuating the problems they experience vis-à-vis the legal system. Their actions, both before and after a malpractice claim is filed, contribute greatly to the etiology and dynamics of these difficulties. Physicians possess a remarkable naivete regarding the numerous pitfalls within the adversary system that can deeply wound them unless they are prepared to act logically and without emotion. Critical factors include the response to the patient at the time of the confrontation, the reaction when an attorney requests information, the response at the time a summons is served, the deposition testimony, demeanor at the trial, and the trial testimony itself.

The physician has always been led to believe that if he maintained good rapport with his patients, he would not have any medical-legal problems. Obviously, he can minimize the threat of a lawsuit if he develops a good relationship with the patient and takes the time to show concern about her problems. The increasing number of claims, however, reflects that this fact alone will not be an absolute deterrent.

Plaintiff

The plaintiff is the person who is asking for money in a lawsuit. The plaintiff is not always the injured patient. If the patient is a child, the lawsuit may be brought by the child's parents or legal guardian. If the patient is deceased, the action may be brought by the representatives of the estate or next of kin. The two most common reasons plaintiffs go to a lawyer to bring a malpractice action are emotional losses and financial demands.

The greatest source of emotional injury seems to be patients' expectations that medical science has progressed to a sophisticated state in which complications and unexpected results do not happen. Patients who are completely aware and fully informed about known risks and complications still do not expect any of these to happen to them. If an unexpected result occurs, it must be someone else's fault. For example, when a patient is gravely injured or dies, other members of the family direct their frustration and anger at those individuals who are associated with the loss by perceiving (misperceiving) fault.

Under such circumstances, honesty, concern, and education are major deterrents to lawsuits. The claimant who is comforted and receives satisfactory answers to lingering questions may not pursue the matter any further. For those cases that do end up in court, the jury will be influenced by the physician's efforts to comfort, reassure, and candidly explain things during and after the patient's care. The advantage is with the physician who adequately documents his efforts in the record.

Economic incentives also play a major role in the instigation and prosecution of a lawsuit. Some persons bring lawsuits because their own economic losses force them into the legal arena. The impact of major medical bills or the loss of earning capacity upon a person or family can be devastating. Patients are almost certain to go to an attorney when medical care with an unfortunate outcome results in lingering medical bills not covered by insurance. Consumer-oriented patients will turn to a lawyer when any action is taken to collect an obligation that is large or that the patient considers unfair or unearned. Any treatment that interrupts the patient's expected flow of wages increases the pressure to recoup. The physician must be cautious in telling patients how long they can expect to be out of work and whether there are foreseeable risks that may result in longer interruptions.

A few plaintiffs, motivated by revenge or greed, look at lawsuits as an instrumentality for gain. The changing mores of our culture seem to breed or reinforce the notion of profiting without work or effort. Every lawyer has people coming into the office whose sole motivation is the green salve of revenge or the green cushion of compensation. Although the physician can often sense such motivation in his patients, he may never even meet the vindictive or greedy relative who becomes the plaintiff following a bad outcome.

The physician's reaction to and attitude toward the patient-turned-plaintiff is a significant consideration. The physician, surprised or shocked at his patient's apparent change of attitude, must not respond in kind. The consequences of such a reaction can be extremely harmful to the litigation. The most successful approach for the physician to take when he comes in contact with a patient who is bringing a lawsuit is to treat the plaintiff with courtesy and respect, to respond without emotion, and to maintain professional poise.

Plaintiff's Attorney

The plaintiff's attorney is the most aggressive of the fraternity of pure pragmatists. He has to be. He is not paid by the hour. He is paid only if he wins; therefore, he operates strictly on a win-loss basis. The contingency fee system can be extremely lucrative. If he wins a case for his client in court, he will likely receive thirty to fifty percent of the award, plus expenses; and the jury cannot be made aware that he may well receive more money than his injured client.

Although a few attorneys also have their medical degrees, the vast majority have only completed the standard three-year general legal education program. Most, therefore, have no specialized training, no medical knowledge, and no supervised experience that qualifies them to enter the lucrative medical malpractice field. To accommodate their lack of knowledge and experience, some attorneys are attending one- and two-day seminars to learn how to evaluate, file, and pursue such cases. They do not have to totally understand the medical facts. They just have to convince a jury that they do. The timetable for attorney's medical education is a source of frustration to the obstetrician-gynecologist, knowing that it took him at least eight years to become the target.

Some lawyers now advertise to get clients for medical malpractice lawsuits. A recent television advertisement asked listeners who might have a brain-damaged child to consider the cause. While the advertisement suggested that the condition could have been caused by genetics or possibly by drugs ingested during the pregnancy, it advised them not to dismiss the idea that someone else might be to blame. Those listeners who had any questions were told to contact the legal firm whose name appeared on the screen.

The attorney's decision to pursue a medical-legal claim is often based on the emotional appeal that can be made to the jury, rather than on the facts of the case. Defendant-physicians have often made this a simple task. Poor documentation in the medical records allows the attorney to create his own scenario, mold it around the deficient record, and present his own set of facts. The plaintiff's attorney can take a case that appeared cut-and-dried at the outset; and by the time it reaches trial, he has created a scenario that is totally different from what the defendant-doctor recalls, a scenario that is, of course, difficult to defend.

One favorite trick of the plaintiff's attorney is to introduce issues that have no bearing on the alleged injury—red herrings. For instance, he can take a notation or lack thereof from the record, twist it, interpret it in his own way, and make it appear that some malintent or negligent act was associated with it. Although at the end of the trial this issue may not be given to the jury to consider, it has been used to create the subsconcious picture of a physician who was not on top of the situation.

One of the most difficult things for the defendant-doctor to understand in the courtroom drama is that a lawyer does not always tell the whole truth—conveniently omitting what does not directly substantiate his theory of the case. The plaintiff's attorney has a duty to his client to see that his claim is portrayed to the court in as favorable a light as possible. He has no duty to the defendant-doctor. He deals with relative rather than absolute truth. He can tell as much or as little as he likes. He can shade it, manipulate it, or simply ignore it.

The opposing lawyer is an object of great frustration, fear, and hostility for the physician. Such emotions can lead to resentment and anger, causing many physicians consciously or unconsciously to take the attorney on as a personal challenge. Feeling he can outtalk and outmaneuver the plaintiff's lawyer, the physician launches a vigorous attack to salve the wounds inflicted by the lawsuit. In such a battle, the defendant-physician will most often find himself the loser. When an opposing lawyer is challenged, he labors harder, prepares more thoroughly, and works more enthusiastically because he has a renewed personal interest in the litigation.

Vigorous and lengthy cross-examination is a tactic used by the experienced plaintiff's attorney to lower the physician's professional demeanor in front of the jury. The attorney deliberately plans his examination to elicit an angry or irrational response from the physician. If he feels the physician has a volatile nature, he tries to get the physician angry. He attempts to intimidate him without appearing intimidating. The physician becomes tired of listening carefully to questions and of selecting words cautiously in his answers. As the stress builds, the temptation to vent his emotions becomes greater. If the defendant's nature is more passive and fearful, a lengthy cross-examination makes him so weary, so fearful, and so anxious to get off the witness stand that he may appear to agree with almost anything the attorney proposes. The goal of the plaintiff's attorney is accomplished in either case. The defendant-doctor has been cast in the role of either the villain or the incompetent.

The cautious physician knows that in the courtroom he is within the attorney's domain, and his testimony is tempered by caution, reason, judgment, preparation, and knowledge. He is well advised to practice sample cross-examination with his own tutor-lawyer in order to assure that the rules of the game are firmly imbedded before he gets on the witness stand.

Defense Attorney

The importance of the defense attorney's role is difficult to overstate. He must be knowledgeable about the medical facts of the case, carefully investigate and prepare the case, tutor the defendant for the production, assess all factors that may potentially win or lose the case, and make recommendations to the insurance company regarding settlement versus trial. However, because the defense attorney is assigned his role in the medical-legal drama by the physician's insurance company, his reputation, ability, and experience are often unknown quantities to the defendant-doctor at the outset. Such casting can place the defense attorney in a somewhat difficult position—although his prime duty may be to the physician-client, he is the chief advisor to both the defendant and the insurance company during the course of litigation.

Preparing for the medical-legal production needs to be a joint effort between the physician and attorney. They must be able to communicate well and to feel comfortable with each other. In order to work well together, the physician must keep his mind open to being legally educated as well as counseled, and the attorney must appreciate the defendant-doctor's range of emotions at having to defend his professional integrity in a hostile, adversarial arena.

When the defendant-doctor first meets with his attorney, he should use both the medical records and his personal recollections to recount everything that he recalls about the specific case. His interpretation of the records and his recollections should not change from initial meeting to deposition or from deposition to trial. Cases have been settled or lost simply because the defendant suddenly changed his personal recollections of events surrounding the alleged negligent action. Although the changes in his story may have nothing to do with the alleged injury, they may be devastating to his credibility.

The physician should provide continued medical input to his attorney throughout the discovery period. Such input may offer new insight into the entire action. Unexpected or unforeseen weaknesses may arise that warrant expert opinion and scientific data to negate. New strengths may be found that could effect a complete and positive change of direction for the defense.

The defense attorney should keep the physician actively participating in the case so that he understands exactly what is going to occur. For example, one often misunderstood aspect of the attorney's investigation and preparation is his need to explore the case from all angles, which involves talking with other physicians in the specialty. Keeping the defendant informed will assure him that the attorney is not going behind his back and that all cases have weak points which need to be uncovered so that the discovery period does not extend into courtroom surprises.

Defendant-doctors often have difficulty dealing with their assigned defense attorneys. If a physician feels uncomfortable with the attorney or feels uneasy about how the case is being handled, he may wish to hire his own personal attorney to monitor the course of the lawsuit. Defense attorneys likewise often have difficulty dealing with physicians who fail to see shortcomings in their own cases. The physician who believes he was absolutely right often fails to recognize factors that need to be considered before going to trial. The attorney knows that simply because the physician may have been completely correct in his judgments regarding the medical treatment does not always mean the case can be won in the courtroom.

At the end of the discovery period, the defense attorney must evaluate all factors that could potentially win or lose the lawsuit:

- status of the medical records (well documented or poorly documented);
- gravity of the injury and the potential loss;
- plaintiff's appearance and credibility;
- defendant's appearance and credibility;
- ability and experience of plaintiff's attorney;
- expert witnesses' appearance and credibility;
- trial judge assigned to case;
- locale in which case is to be tried; and
- caliber of jurors available in specific locale.

Once the decision is made to proceed to trial, the defense attorney must carefully prepare the defendant-doctor for the final production. Besides addressing the specifics of the case, the attorney needs to explain the procedures, tactics, and rules that can have a significant influence in the legal setting. For instance, the defendant-doctor needs to understand that he will be under constant observation throughout the trial and that his unspoken role is as important as when he is on the witness stand. Such factors as his dress (conservative or extravagant, neat or rumpled) and his demeanor (attentive or bored, concerned or angry) are important in determining whether the judge and jury cast him as a villain or a hero, a professional or an incompetent. In addition, the attorney can help the defendant-doctor learn how to communicate positively in the courtroom by advising him about the legal trickery he will likely encounter and how best to handle himself during such adverse moments. At all times, the defendant-doctor must appear to be in personal command. He needs to understand that the defense goal is to provide the jury with the lasting image of a concerned and competent physician, one who is both caring and careful.

Insurance Carrier

The insurance carrier is a silent participant in the medical-legal drama, but one who can pull the curtain during any act of the production because it holds the purse strings. Once a claim is reported or filed, the carrier is represented by a claims manager, whose job, of necessity, is to continually evaluate potential win-loss ratios. However, long before a claim is filed and the drama begins, the physician himself purchases a professional liability insurance policy and, thus, decides which insurance company will play this critical role.

Most physicians purchase their professional liability insurance from either a physician-owned insurance company or a commercial carrier.* These companies sell three kinds of professional liability insurance. The *claims made policy* only covers claims that are reported or filed during the time period the policy is in effect. The *occurrence policy* covers any claim made regarding an incident that occurred during the year the policy was in effect. In order to extend coverage after the time period covered by a claims made policy, physicians must purchase a *tail policy,* which essentially converts the claims made policy into an occurrence policy.

The premiums that physicians pay for these policies are, by almost everyone's standards, outrageously high and still increasing. However, the daily paper answers the question why. Settlements and jury awards, especially in obstetric cases, seem to have leaped completely out of bounds. Even if the claims manager concludes that a case is winnable, juries are unpredictable, and the case may be lost and an overwhelming amount awarded. Fear of the unknown verdict often effects a settlement that is out of proportion to the liability. Each large settlement or jury award only increases the likelihood that the next one will be larger.

Most physicians are opposed to having spurious cases settled based

---

* For a discussion of other sources, such as self-insurance and captive insurance companies, see Chapter 17, Risk Management and Loss Prevention in the Hospital.

on the argument that it would cost the insurance carrier more to defend the case than settle it. To settle such a case not only is a subtle admission of guilt, but it also puts an unfavorable mark on the physician's record. A pattern of settling spurious cases may encourage plaintiffs' attorneys to accept and pursue a large number of cases in anticipation of making a substantial income from a large number of small settlements. However, physicians often cannot prohibit the carrier from settling such a case because state laws or the terms of the insurance policy allow the carrier to settle cases without the physician's permission. Many physicians believe their consent ought to be required before a case is settled since the outcome of a case affects their insurance premiums. They believe they have a right to the same informed consent they are required to give their patients—that they are entitled to know what their choices are, what the risks are from the proposed approach, and what alternatives are available. With an increasing number of claims being filed and the decision about settlement being made by the insurance carrier, the physician may find himself in the catch-22 situation of having these unfavorable marks on his record resulting in the cancellation of his professional liability coverage.

In addition to the controversy over settlements, professional liability insurance and policy carriers can introduce as many headaches as they solve. For example, physicians often fear that if they report every potential claim, their insurance coverage may eventually be dropped; yet, early reporting of potential claims is important. The physician should be aware that any information given to the insurance company (written or tape recorded) can be discovered by the plaintiff in a subsequent action. The information in these communications must match other records or the physician has impeached himself. Therefore, the physician is well advised to give details only to a designated attorney, since communications with one's attorney are considered work product and cannot be discovered. Physicians are also concerned about the possibility of an insurance carrier deciding to take a case to trial when the award could exceed the physician's policy limits. In such a case, the physician may need his own attorney to negotiate with the insurance company. The physician who wants the case settled should make those feelings known in writing; then if the insurance company does proceed to trial and there is a verdict against the physician that exceeds his coverage, he will have some legal recourse. Another area of concern centers around punitive damages, which are not covered by professional liability insurance. Although punitive damages have been extremely rare in the past, a recent Kansas jury awarded $15 million to a plaintiff, the majority of which was for punitive damages. If the decision is approved by the court, the obstetricians involved in the case would be personally responsible for over $1 million of that amount.

Most physicians do not become disenchanted with their insurance carriers until after a claim is filed. At that time, it is too late. Professional liability insurance is an ethical and sometimes a legal imperative that requires the thoughtful consideration given to any major purchase, i.e., the physician should know exactly what he is buying before he does so.

- He should know if the insurance carrier he is considering is financially stable. Financial reports are generally a matter of public record. He should also know if his particular state has established insolvency or guarantee funds designed to protect him if the company should become insolvent.
- He should understand the exact type of policy he purchases and make sure the coverage fits his own needs and expectations. He may wish to have an attorney review the contract.
- The physician should know the company's reputation for quality of service rendered. He can ask fellow physicians if they are satisfied that the company responds in a prompt, efficient, and courteous manner.
- He needs to determine the names and reputations of law firms in the area that the company uses. He should be aware that some law firms will not work with certain insurance companies because the hourly wage is so low.
- The physician needs to know the management philosophy of the carrier and determine whether this philosophy fits his own. For example, he should know the company's attitude regarding cost control, since it is desirable to have a claims department that does not settle claims completely lacking merit simply to avoid legal expense.

In mid-1984, representatives of ACOG told a congressional committee that sixty percent of all obstetrician-gynecologists in the nation have been sued, twenty percent of them three or more times.[1] These statistics should help the obstetrician-gynecologist understand the importance of making an informed choice about his insurance coverage. The purchase of professional liability insurance may be one of the most expensive and most important decisions the physician will ever make because it affects him both professionally and financially.

Medical Experts

Before a lawsuit may proceed to trial, the plaintiff usually must have an expert opinion of medical deviation, and these opinions must come from members of the medical profession. Medical experts espousing either side of a dispute may not be difficult to find. As plaintiffs' attorneys are presently advertising for clients, so some physicians are actively soliciting business as medical experts. These expert witnesses come from many quarters.

The *credible expert* is the most difficult to find. He does not need to solicit business. If he testifies for the defense, the medical community loves him. If he testifies for the plaintiff, the plaintiff community holds him in high esteem, and physicians view him with suspicion. He is medically wise, thorough, fair, and honest. Because he has these special qualities, he may be requested to be an expert so often that he soon burns out. Evaluating a claim is tedious and time consuming, and participating in depositions and trials is much more traumatic than treating patients. However, such an expert witness educates the court properly and is extremely valuable to the system.

The *professional expert* does little else than analyze and evaluate claims and give expert opinion and testimony. Some of these witnesses routinely provide testimony only for the plaintiff or only for the defense. Such witnesses lose credibility because fairness and honesty are never one-sided.

The *flip-over expert* gives testimony for whoever gets to him first, plaintiff or defense. One such witness recently found he had given opinions for both sides in the same case. He obviously had to withdraw from the case. These last two types of witness are vulnerable at the time of trial since their position on an issue often changes from case to case. The attorney who does his homework will review all of a witness's prior testimony and will be able to impeach such a witness's credibility.

The *ivory tower expert* practices only in academia or in large institutions. Many of these experts routinely pass negative judgment on physicians who practice with limited facilities and personnel. Although basic standards should apply across the board, specialized emergency responses cannot be dealt with in the same manner in all settings.

The *plaintiff's scenario expert* bases his opinion on a written statement that the plaintiff gave to her attorney at the outset of a legal action. This statement and the attorney's supporting scenario are discussed with the expert before he has had an opportunity to examine the medical records. Although the actual records may not substantiate the plaintiff's scenario, this type of expert molds his opinion around the preconception. A plaintiff's statement should be considered as only one part of the total record. Obviously, a patient who is pursuing legal action has many hostile feelings regarding what she perceives was inappropriate care. In some instances, she may be right; in others, however, the perceptions of a medically untrained mind may be in error or drastically altered by the time attorney contact is made.

The *omnipotent expert* gives opinions that reflect a level of perfection that he himself does not achieve in practice. One such expert wrote that the failure to diagnose a breech presentation was regrettable but understandable because of the patient's obesity. At trial, he testified that failure to diagnose the breech was unjustifiable; yet when queried about his own practice, the expert acknowledged that he, too, had failed to diagnose the presentation on prior occasions.

The *fill-in-the-blanks expert* supplies the missing information when asked to review incomplete or poorly documented records. Although a plaintiff's attorney may send the expert only those records he wants him to see, it is the expert's responsibility to request those records needed to get the total picture of the alleged deviation. If the records are poorly documented, the expert should not assume that the blank spaces reveal negligence.

The *I've-got-just-a-minute expert* spends little time reviewing the record and gives a hasty opinion. It is quite impossible to thoroughly evaluate all records of a case in a short period of time. An opinion based on hasty initial impressions might be drastically altered if the expert would closely explore and consider the total historical data.

The *trapped ego expert* examines the record and sends his opinion to the attorney, citing the basis for that opinion. He later realizes he misinterpreted the record. Instead of acknowledging he made a mistake, he then proceeds to find a way to defend his original opinion. His testimony may not be one hundred percent believable, but he has allowed the case to go to the jury.

The *I'm-your-everything expert* evaluates claims, gives opinions, and testifies about a field in which he is not knowledgeable. The most obvious example occurs in brain-damaged children cases. This expert speaks not only to the standard of obstetric care, but also gives his opinion regarding causation. He usually has no knowledge or training in neurology, does not know what or where the exact injury is, or is unaware of whether any specific diagnostic testing for etiology has been attempted.

All those who would be medical experts should remember that they may become defendants in the future. In a restatement of the golden rule, they should evaluate each case in the same manner that they would expect their own to be evaluated.

Judge

Another of the participants in the courtroom drama is the trial judge. The judge interprets and rules on points of law as they apply to the issues that arise during the trial. At the end of the trial, he gives instructions to the jury, advising them about what the law is and how they are supposed to apply it to the facts in this specific case.

When the trial begins, the defendant-doctor views the courtroom as a revered setting in which truth will at long last out. He respects the judge as someone above partiality or bias. In fact, many physicians believe that decisions in medical malpractice cases would be more desirable if they were made by judges, who they consider to be less apt to let emotions sway their decisions. They assume that judges are more sympathetic because they come from the same achievement-oriented segment of society and understand what it means to be a professional.

However, judges, just like doctors, are not gods; they are people who come in all different sizes, shapes, and forms. They have no medical training and are likely to be as naive as each juror about the specific medical facts of a case. Some judges are elected; some are appointed. Since most judges were in practice before reaching the bench, any bias for the plaintiff or the defense usually depends on the type of law they practiced. They may be liberal or conservative. Some judges are very intelligent; some are not. Some have more inherent ability than others to apply the law. Some judges pay close attention to the trial proceedings; some doze off from time to time. All judges have their own expectations, their own patterns of logic, and their own prejudices.

The judge is an influential courtroom player who pays close attention to the defendant, even when he is not testifying. He, like the jurors, forms conclusions about the defendant based on how the defendant dresses, his ability to communicate, and his total demeanor. Although he is to be impartial and unbiased, his feelings are often passed on to the jury by his facial expressions, his responses to the attorneys, and the rulings he makes.

Each judge is unique, and each is extremely powerful. The judge controls the course of the trial much like a referee in an important sports event. He makes good calls and bad calls without the benefit of instant replay, and his rulings often play an important role in determining the winner.

Jury

The jury is the audience in this courtroom drama. These individuals—traditionally, six in federal court or twelve in district court—have their own distinct personalities, their own level of education, their own pattern of thinking, and their own prejudices. They bring with them their own unique expectations of the medical profession. While the judge is supposed to apply the law to the subject, the trial jury is the legal determiner of the facts. After the judge gives the jurors instructions at the end of the trial, they are then given free rein to determine what actually happened, what the standard of care required be done, and what award or damages, if any, should be made.

The jury system has existed for centuries. Jurors were once much like witnesses. They were called because they had knowledge of the facts. Today, a prospective juror with special knowledge about the case is often rejected out of hand.

Lawyers generally approve of juries, believing the diversity of people assures that an average balance of common sense is applied in the case. A jury-tried case avoids the individual biases of any one judge, although a jury may be pressured by emotional presentations.

Physicians are not convinced that their actions are being judged by a "jury of their peers." They are concerned about a system that requires laymen to become medically educated enough to make technical judgments about sophisticated medical decisions and actions that it took them years of specialty training to achieve. The courtroom is a poor setting for a medical education. The medically untrained plaintiff's attorney tells the jury what the medical facts are; the medically untrained defense attorney then tells them what he perceives the facts to be; and the medical experts argue over which story is correct. Truth is elusive, and the jury must decide whose version is more believable. Truth then becomes a matter of opinion.

Many physicians do not know quite how to communicate with the jury. Some physicians believe that juries are composed of ignorant people who do not, cannot, and will not understand the basic principles. The attitude of a physician who talks down to the jury and uses a grade school vocabulary in explaining things is generally perceived by the jury as offensive. On the other hand, the physician who bombards the jury with complicated, jargon-filled sentences paints an equally offensive picture of arrogance. Both extremes are equally bad. Jurors do not react well to being treated as though they are as ignorant as they might actually be. At the same time, they must understand the facts in the case in order to intelligently weigh the issues. Such balanced communication requires the preparation and thought accorded to any major presentation. The preparation of the script, the choice of words, and the exercise of communication skills are just as important in the courtroom as they are in any other drama.

Most jurors feel it is their duty to search for the truth and to see that justice is served. The medical-legal drama becomes much like a mystery awaiting solution. Each juror waits daily for additional clues, for each wishes to solve the mystery and to understand exactly how and when the alleged injury occurred. In some cases, exact etiologies are not known. However, plaintiff's counsel and experts tell the jury that they, of course, know the exact etiology. When defense counsel and experts truthfully counter that the exact etiology is unknown, juries often perceive this as an attempt to avoid the truth, to cover an action that could have prevented the outcome. They subconsciously feel that they must have an answer to justify the difficult decision they will be asked to make at the end of the trial.

During the production, the jurors are often confused by attorneys' objections and the trial judge's rulings. For example, they do not understand the technicalities involved in determining what testimony can and cannot be admitted or what it means to disregard testimony they have already heard.

Although most jurors have common sense, their decisions are subconsciously and emotionally molded by many factors, many of which have nothing to do with the facts in the case. They constantly observe the demeanor of the defendant and all of his interactions with his attorney, the plaintiff, the plaintiff's attorney, the expert witnesses, the judge, and the jury itself. They search for clues in all of the other players' interactions with each other. They are especially curious about nonparticipating parties present in the courtroom. Often the appearance, demeanor, and expression of the physician's spouse, office assistants, relatives, or friends may influence them.

By the time the judge gives instructions, most jurors have already formed an opinion. Those who have some hesitation or reservations are usually then influenced by the reasoning of the other jurors. The final verdict reflects the composite judgment of the group. Some of the jurors will believe they have discovered the truth and that justice has been served. Some are simply relieved they can return to their normal routine. Half of the courtroom players will agree with the decision; the other half will not. However, this panel has reached an opinion that satisfies the court's purposes. In the courtroom, truth and justice have very broad boundaries.

Guidelines

The physician who gets involved in a lawsuit should discuss the case at the earliest point with his lawyer. He should make sure that the lawyer understands the problems as the physician sees them. The physician should review textbooks and medical articles on the subject. He should make sure that the defense lawyer has probed for the weaknesses in the case. The physician who takes the attitude that there is no malpractice and therefore no legal exposure makes a gross mistake. *Every case has weaknesses!* The physician must be prepared to keep the opposition from capitalizing on them. The physician should make sure that the defense lawyer has talked with other physicians who have differing viewpoints. The physician must not be offended if his colleagues criticize him, because the defense lawyer must know exactly what the weaknesses are in the case in order to formulate the defense. After the weaknesses are recognized, then it is important to determine whether or not the impact of these weaknesses can be avoided. Even if the physician was negligent, there may well be no causal relationship to the injury for which the patient is suing. Often there are preexisting illnesses or predispositions that are crucial to the case, and the physician should make sure that the patient's previous medical records are obtained and carefully reviewed not only by himself but by independent, objective evaluators.*

At the deposition, the opposition lawyer asks the physician questions that probe into the reasons for his actions. Before that deposition, the physician should have carefully reviewed the medical records. He should know what the medical textbooks say on the subject. The physician may find that these textbooks disagree with his approach; in order to be prepared, he must determine in advance whether there is more than one school of thought on the subject. He may well find that equally authoritative sources have recommended an approach similar to his, and it is important for both the physician and his attorney to recognize that there are two schools and to be aware of the differences.

---

* See Chapter 15, Claims Analysis, for a further discussion.

The physician must also know the standards of his professional organizations. However, ACOG's book of standards specifically states,

> *the standards set down here are presented as recommendations and general guidelines rather than as a body of rigid rules. They are intended to be adapted to many different situations, taking into account the needs and resources particular to the locality, the institution or type of practice. Variation and innovation which demonstrably improve the quality of patient care are to be encouraged rather than restricted* [p. ii].[2]

Even so, he must be aware of what those standards are, as well as be prepared to explain and interpret those standards as well as his actions vis-à-vis those standards. The physician must know his hospital's rules, regulations, bylaws, or standing orders that require particular actions be taken at certain times. If the physician deviated from those standards, he should be prepared to show that those standards are obsolete, are not applicable, or are not relevant to this case.

Before his deposition, the physician must carefully go over the rules of deposition taking with his lawyer.* Not only must he understand them, but he must be prepared to cope with them on a practical basis. Many attorneys make it a practice to harass and intimidate their own clients with sample cross-examinations in order to make sure that they get the worst from their own counsel rather than from the opposition. This type of preparation well in advance gives the physician the opportunity to correct the mistakes that could make a major difference in the outcome of the litigation.

Conclusion

When you receive your summons or subpoena, may you remember all the different actors and the parts they play. You now know how many factors that are totally unrelated to the true technical merits of the claim can have striking effects on the outcome. Your appearance, your demeanor, and your actions may be just as important as the issue of fault. You also understand that those who conduct this legal orchestration have an excellent, finely tuned system to bring legal certainty into our lives. Legal certainty is different from justice. As students are told as they begin their legal training, if they wanted justice, they should have gone to a seminary.

---

* See Chapter 8, Testifying in Medical-Legal Cases, for a further discussion.

References

1. American Medical Association Special Task Force on Professional Liability and Insurance. Professional liability in the '80s: report 1. Chicago: American Medical Association, 1984.
2. American College of Obstetricians and Gynecologists. Standards for obstetric-gynecologic services, ed 5. Washington, DC: Author, 1982.

Chapter 7

Participating in the Legal Process:
A Guide for the Defendant-Physician
Walter A. Oleniewski

Medical malpractice is unfairly viewed by many as the bane of the medical profession and the boon of the legal profession. However, I believe that everyone will admit that there are times when an injured party deserves compensation because his injuries were sustained through no fault of his own and were avoidable. Accidents that happen in operating rooms are no more intentional than automobile accidents that occur on highways. In the vast majority of medical malpractice cases, the respective parties to the litigation are well-meaning with the plaintiffs believing that they are entitled to the compensation they seek and with the defendants believing that they have properly treated the patients to the best of their ability. To ferret out the meritorious cases and to discourage the frivolous ones requires the cooperation of both the medical and legal professions.

This need for cooperation is an ongoing process which begins when the physician first becomes aware that he will be involved in a medical malpractice case, whether it arises as a result of treatment rendered a patient or consultation from a referring colleague or whether he will be called upon as an expert witness to review the care given by other medical providers. In addition, the cooperation must be candid. Too frequently during the final steps of preparing a malpractice lawsuit for trial, an attorney will learn new information relevant to the case that his client-physician possessed but did not disclose to him. Just as a physician expects his patients to follow his advice and to cooperate in recommended therapy, an attorney expects the same of his client. An attorney must have his client's trust in order to ensure that all relevant matters necessary for the thorough preparation of the defense are given appropriate consideration. Any surprises should occur well in advance of the trial so that they may be properly assessed and countered. Surprises during the trial may prove to be not only embarrassing to the physician but a detrimental influence on the outcome of the litigation.

The participation of medical specialists is an essential ingredient in practically all medical malpractice litigation. Attorneys generally can neither establish the existence of malpractice nor disprove an allegation of substandard medical practice without the testimony of medical experts. Opinions expressed in letters, journals, articles, or textbooks are generally not admissible evidence because they are hearsay and the authors are unavailable for cross-examination. The physician who was involved in the plaintiff-patient's treatment will be unable to avoid participation in the litigation; the physician who was not involved in the patient's treatment and who is called upon to serve as an expert witness or consultant to the attorney is not required to participate in the litigation. However, every physician's concerns about the malpractice crisis demand that the time and energy necessary be devoted to providing a sound, impartial basis for the judgment that must be made by individuals who are unfamiliar with medicine. When conscientious practitioners decline to participate in malpractice litigation, professional witnesses who derive much of their income from testifying will continue to impart their predilections without adequate challenge.

Discovery

Although each state and the federal government have their own laws and judicial structure, every jurisdiction in the United States recognizes the adversary system and permits recourse to some form of trial for the resolution of the issues involved in an allegation of medical malpractice. There are certain preliminary matters, which attorneys refer to as *discovery,* that are intended to permit each opponent to discover information concerning his adversary's case. If carefully conducted, discovery eliminates all unnecessary issues and enables the litigants to either settle the matter or present it for trial in an efficient, effective manner, without any surprises. While there may be variations from one state to another, they all generally recognize the five types of pretrial discovery: (1) interrogatories, (2) depositions, (3) requests for admissions, (4) document production, and (5) physical and mental examinations. Through these vehicles, attorneys can assess the strengths and weaknesses of their respective clients' positions. Since the physician's participation in these aspects of discovery varies, their significance should be understood.

Interrogatories

Interrogatories, which are a set of written questions prepared by parties to the litigation and addressed to another party in the same lawsuit, are designed primarily to elicit facts and to identify relevant materials and witnesses. They are not addressed to witnesses who are not a party to the lawsuit. For example, interrogatories addressed to a plaintiff might seek basic biographical information, work history, medical history, and the extent of injuries relating to the litigation, including costs, dates, and places of treatment. They would further seek to identify the expert witnesses to be called and the substance of each expert's opinion. The defendant-physician may be called upon to respond to interrogatories requiring a description of the events and his recollections surrounding the incidents that gave rise to the litigation as well as the names of expert witnesses who will testify on his behalf and documents that will be offered into evidence.

An attorney sends the interrogatory to the attorney who represents his opponent, and consultation between attorney and client is appropriate in drafting the answers which must be returned within a set number of days, usually thirty. Since answers to interrogatories may be used during the trial, their content is most important. Physicians who do not appreciate the significance of this preliminary paperwork may come to regret an interrogatory answer that contradicts their trial testimony.

Frequently, an interrogatory will ask a party to identify his expert witnesses and to provide summaries of their testimony. In answering the interrogatory, the party, rather than speculating, should contact each expert witness and ask them to supply the information necessary to answer it. The expert witnesses' responses are crucial, since they may serve as the cornerstone for the entire defense.

Interrogatories are widely used. They have an advantage over oral depositions in that they are less expensive and may require the party responding to them to conduct some inquiry and research before preparing an answer. However, they lack the flexibility of oral depositions, limiting the extent of their usefulness.

Oral Depositions

An oral deposition is the statement of a witness under oath, taken in question-and-answer form as it would be in court. The attorneys representing the parties to the litigation are present and participate in the examination and cross-examination of the witness. The testimony is recorded verbatim and subsequently transcribed.

Oral depositions are the most widely used of the discovery devices. While most courts provide a method for taking the discovery deposition of a witness by written questions, it is rarely used because of the same inflexibility associated with interrogatories. The greatest advantage of an oral deposition is that it allows attorneys the opportunity to probe a witness, to require immediate, on-the-spot answers to questions, and to frame additional questions in response to answers that are given. The greatest disadvantage of an oral deposition is the expense.

In recent years, videotape depositions have become widespread, especially when it is anticipated that the deponent will not be present at the trial. A videotape deposition is conducted in a manner similar to trial testimony, with the exception that a judge is not present to rule on objections, and may appear to be stilted since it lacks the spontaneity involved in responding to courtroom events. However, a videotape permits the judge and jury to view the overall demeanor of the deponent whose testimony would otherwise be a written transcript that would give no opportunity to weigh the credibility of the speaker.

The usual purpose of an oral deposition is not to preserve testimony for trial but to discover what the opponent's witnesses may testify to if they are called as witnesses during the trial. Although a discovery deposition is generally conducted in an informal setting, a court reporter is present, administers an oath to the witness, and then records the examination of the witness in its entirety. The attorney conducting the deposition will also be present as well as any other parties and their attorneys who wish to be present. The importance of a deposition cannot be overemphasized. A witness must be as prepared for his discovery deposition as for his trial testimony. While the deposition is nominally one for discovery purposes, it may be used as evidence in the trial, either to substitute for a witness who is genuinely unavailable or to impeach his credibility during cross-examination.

Credibility is a critical factor—one which an attorney wishes to preserve in his witnesses and to undercut in the witnesses of his opposition. An oral deposition sets the stage for an attack on the credibility of an opposition witness during the trial.

Each attorney develops his own style of conducting depositions. First, the location of the deposition must be determined. While it might be convenient to depose a witness in the attorney's own office, a deposition taken in the physician's office enables the attorney to observe the textbooks and journals that the physician most likely relies upon as authoritative. The attorney may obtain copies of some of these published materials to compromise the witness's credibility if they condone practices contrary to those espoused by the physician. Second, the date and time of a deposition are usually set by the mutual convenience of the attorneys. For the most part, however, deposition dates are flexible, even when the witness has been served with a subpoena, and any questions that arise about a scheduled conflict should be discussed with the appropriate attorney. It is foolhardy for attorneys to schedule depositions without determining the doctor's availability since his ability to devote his full attention will be seriously hampered if the deposition is taken during an inordinately inconvenient time.

In preparation for giving a deposition, the physician should review only those records, reports, opinions, depositions, statements, and other materials necessary either to support the opinion he will express or to recall his own participation in the examination and treatment of the patient. It is unnecessary and unwise to review everything that has transpired in the litigation. As a general rule, the more the physician knows or appears to know about the case, the longer the deposition. If in doubt of the extent of review, the witness should consult the attorney, who may have additional information for the witness's consideration. For example, a named party to the litigation should review any interrogatory answers previously given. Preparation for a deposition is essential, and the witness should insist on spending time with the attorney to discuss the likely areas of inquiry and generally to be aware of what to expect and how to react. No amount of preparation for the trial itself will negate the damage done by an ill-prepared comment made at the deposition. When conducting a discovery deposition, attorneys normally seek to have the deponent do most of the talking. Questions that are asked will likely be open-ended—aimed at getting a full, complete explanation—as opposed to a leading question which effectively suggests the answer to the witness. Open-ended questions are replete with such well-used phrases as "Tell us what happened next.

Please go on. Is there anything else? What do you recall?" Typical cross-examination questions frequently start with such phraseology as, "Do you agree, Dr. X, that . . . ? You will concede, won't you, that . . . . Isn't it true that . . . ?" Attorneys are trained to not ask a witness the question "why" during a trial, especially during cross-examination, unless they know the answer or do not care what the answer is. The witness has an opportunity to explain his answer if asked "why," and if the attorney does not know the answer, a surprise comment during the trial may have an adverse effect on his case. However, the same comment in a discovery deposition can put the attorney on notice that he will have to prepare his own case to overcome the comment at the trial. Thus, during discovery depositions where the purpose is to find out what the witness knows, "why" questions are the rule rather than the exception.

Attorneys try to find expert witnesses for their case from many sources, including friends, relatives, colleagues, medical schools, recognized authorities, publications, and opposing medical experts during their depositions. Credibility is the major product to be sold at the trial; therefore, if one witness concedes that another individual is more of an authority or is more credible, then the latter individual will more likely be viewed as having the correct answer or opinion. As an example, during a discovery deposition, an obstetrician may be asked for the identities of the leading practitioners in his own field, either locally or nationally, or the identity of a consultant he would call upon if he had a particularly difficult obstetrical problem. Likewise, his instructors from medical school or during his residency program may also serve as potential expert witnesses. If any of these individuals can then be called as an expert witness, they will clearly be seen as more authoritative and more credible than the obstetrician who initially revealed their identities and who has already indicated that they may be more knowledgeable than himself.

In the same vein, witnesses are asked for the names of textbooks and journals that they consider to be authoritative. It is difficult to avoid relying upon some materials as authoritative. However, unless the witness is thoroughly familiar with a publication, it is permissible and advisable for the witness to qualify his answer by indicating that he may not agree with the publication in its entirety. The witness is entitled to disagree with a recognized author if there is a sound, scientific basis. Accordingly, if an obstetrician is directly asked about a textbook that is universally recognized as authoritative in his field of specialty, he would not be credible if he declined to recognize it as a learned treatise in that medical specialty. However, unless he is familiar and in agreement with all of the material relevant to the case in controversy that is contained in the text, any acknowledgment of its authoritativeness should be qualified by indicating a disagreement or less than complete acceptance of all of the book's contents. The witness may qualify his acceptance in a general comment without reference to any particular passages from the publication unless he is directed to a specific section of the text. If that occurs, the witness may ask to examine the text before expressing agreement or disagreement.

A bibliography of a witness's publications and professional presentations also provides an excellent opportunity to determine whether the physician's practice is consistent with his conduct or testimony, and inquiry concerning them may frequently occur in a deposition. Similarly, any speeches or lectures dealing with the relevant subject matter may present an opportunity to measure the witness's consistency.

On occasion an expert witness testifies beyond his recognized field of competence. As a general rule, a physician should not render medical treatment (except in an emergency) or provide expert medical testimony beyond the areas in which he would be called upon as a consultant or for which he would be granted hospital staff privileges. If professional peers would not ask for an individual's opinion or allow him to practice in a specialty field, the jury can hardly be expected to accept this person's opinions in those areas. Depositions serve an essential role in delineating the limits of an expert's area of competence.

In the deposition, the witness should be aware of the following points. It is permissible for the witness to speak to his attorney in preparation for the deposition. If asked whether the case has been discussed with anyone, the witness should be truthful in his response. Most attorney-client conversations are privileged, and the witness will not have to respond to questions that violate any privilege.* When asked a question that is unclear or that requires additional information to clarify it, the witness is entitled to ask to have it repeated or to state his difficulty in understanding it. The witness should take a short pause between ques-

---

* Attorney-client conversations are generally privileged. This condition does not necessarily extend to all other conversations with an attorney. Therefore, if the physician has a conversation with an attorney who does not represent him or who may depose him, such privilege may not apply. The physician should raise the question of privilege with the attorney during deposition preparation to avoid being surprised or embarrassed during the deposition.

tion and answer and then devote enough time to present a complete response. The witness who does not know or remember should so state and should not guess at the answer. Furthermore, the witness should leave his temper at home. The only purpose served by a show of anger is to prolong the deposition and have an emotional response affect an otherwise considered answer.

Finally, the witness should be aware of the *stare* tactic used by lawyers. In any kind of conversation, an individual is naturally inclined to provide additional information, to go beyond an answer already considered to be complete, simply because the party seeking the answer stares at you. Every student experiences this tendency whenever a teacher calls upon him and then continues to stare at the student upon completion of the answer. In this uncomfortable situation, the natural tendency is to think the answer is incomplete and that additional information is necessary. This temptation should be resisted, and assuming the answer was complete, the witness should be aware of and ignore the stare tactic.

Requests for Admission

Every case involves many facts, both disputed and undisputed. Some of them will necessarily be proven by the testimony presented during the trial as part of a persuasive development of the case, and it would hardly be an effective tool to stipulate or admit the lack of dispute concerning matters that would best be presented through live testimony. However, to avoid the expense, time, and inconvenience of proving every fact in a trial, courts have established procedures by which one party may request his adversary to admit the genuineness of certain facts and of certain documents that are not at issue and that will not be contested during the trial. Employing these procedures eliminates surprise and expedites the trial by disposing of the tedious proof of all facts presented. Requests for admission cannot be served on a witness, but rather must be served on an opposing party. Thus, if requests are submitted, they will generally ask the party to admit that certain statements constitute fact, for example, (1) "Jane Smith underwent a caesarean section at General Hospital, Kenosha, Wisconsin, on January 7, 1981" and (2) "the left hypogastric artery was severed at that operation." The physician should cooperate with the attorney in determining which requests for admission about the patient's treatment should be admitted.

Document Production

Most courts permit litigants to have access to relevant documents regardless of who might have custody of them. There may, however, be some limitations on the access, such as permission only to inspect them, to copy them, or to take custody of them. In a medical malpractice suit, the obvious documents that are critical to the litigation are the medical records. These records include any type of document, material, or specimen that reflects some memorialization of the treatment rendered, including x-rays, electronic tracing data such as electrocardiograms (EKGs) or fetal heart tracings, and slides.

Document production can occur in one of three ways. They may be produced (1) voluntarily or through the compulsory processes of (2) a motion to produce or (3) a subpoena duces tecum. The motion to produce will ordinarily be granted only against the parties to the litigation, and the motion will identify certain documents or categories of documents that are desired for inspection, custody, and/or duplication. A subpoena duces tecum compels a witness to appear for a deposition and to simultaneously produce the documents designated in the subpoena. Often an attorney is only interested in obtaining a copy of the medical records from a reluctant physician and will forego a deposition if the records are produced prior to the scheduled deposition. However, the physician who is served with a subpoena duces tecum should consult with his attorney, particularly since it may be necessary to prepare for a deposition.

Physical and Mental Examinations

Since the severity and extent of the patient's injuries are a central focus in a medical malpractice case, the genuineness of the complaint and prognosis of the injury are of concern to the parties. Every jurisdiction has some provision to require a plaintiff to undergo an examination by a doctor selected by either the defendant or the court regarding the injuries that are the subject of the suit. The extent of the examination may have to be set by the court, which generally will not compel a plaintiff to submit to invasive techniques. However, in severe cases, such as profound cerebral palsy or paralysis and associated ailments, the examination may be conducted in a hospital with several medical specialists conducting necessary consultations over several days. The selection of the physician who will conduct the examination of the plaintiff is critical to the final evaluation of the injuries and to the monetary value that may be placed on them should a settlement be considered or a trial be unavoidable.

Trial

Overview

As with any trial, thorough preparation, which includes an understanding of the facts of the case and the law applicable to the matter in issue, is essential. The major focus of a medical malpractice trial is on the confrontation of medical expert testimony. If the case is to be decided by a jury rather than by a judge, the trial process begins with the selection of a jury. The role of the judge is always to rule on issues of law and to determine the law that is applicable and that controls the issues in the litigation. The jury resolves factual issues and applies the controlling law to the facts in order to arrive at a decision about both negligence and monetary value.

After jury selection, counsel for both plaintiff and defendant will make their opening statements. Testimony will then commence with the plaintiff presenting all of his witnesses and eliciting their testimony through direct examination, with the defendant's counsel cross-examining each of the witnesses. The judge may also ask questions; and on a very limited basis, a juror may be permitted to write down a question and submit it to the judge who will determine whether it will be propounded to the witness. Upon the completion of all of his witnesses' testimony and the introduction of all necessary documentary evidence, the plaintiff will rest his case. At that time, the defendant will ordinarily make a formal motion to the judge to dismiss the case or to direct a verdict for the defendant. In essence, the defense attorney is arguing that he should not be required to produce any evidence because the plaintiff failed to present evidence that would constitute a prima facie case, that is, evidence that in the judgment of the law would be sufficient to entitle the plaintiff to a favorable finding of liability unless the defendant can contradict and overcome it by other evidence. If the judge agrees with the defense attorney, the trial is complete, the jury is discharged, and the defense does not call any witnesses. If the judge is of the opinion that the plaintiff has presented a prima facie case or if the judge wishes to defer a decision on that issue until a later time, the defendant calls all of his witnesses and introduces his documentary evidence.

At the conclusion of the defendant's case, some additional motions may be made by either attorney regarding the sufficiency of the evidence and whether one party is entitled to a favorable judgment from the judge because the law and the facts of the case are so overwhelmingly in his favor that if the matter were submitted to the jury, it could only be resolved by the jury for the one party. Assuming the judge declines to rule in favor of either party, the plaintiff is given a final opportunity to present rebuttal evidence to reply to some of the evidence provided by the defendant. On its conclusion or after the opportunity to present rebuttal evidence has been declined, the attorneys will make their closing arguments, and the judge will instruct the jurors as to the applicable law and the procedure for conducting their deliberations. Most courts require the jury verdict to be unanimous; however, in civil trials, there is a growing number of states where less than a unanimous verdict is permissible.

The average person's knowledge of court proceedings ordinarily comes from television and newspapers. By and large, they are exposed to criminal trials and to the special standard of burden of proof in criminal law—proof beyond a reasonable doubt. In a medical malpractice trial, the burden of proof is that of a preponderance or greater weight of the evidence. Based on one hundred percent, fifty-one percent constitutes a preponderance of the evidence. Accordingly, the burden of proof is not as demanding as in a criminal trial, which requires proof beyond a reasonable doubt; expressed in percentages, it would be into the ninetieth percentile approaching one hundred percent.

Trial Testimony

The most obvious difference between trial testimony and a discovery deposition is the setting. Informality is gone. The judge and courtroom can intimidate even the most seasoned trial attorneys, let alone a first-time witness. Because the physician is unfamiliar with a courtroom and the permissible rules of conduct and evidence, his confidence can be shaken by an aggressive cross-examining attorney—unless he understands the application of the tools of the attorney's trade as well as the attorney's motives and goals.

Direct Examination

Direct examination occurs when a witness is called by an attorney, who wants the witness either to recount his participation in the treatment of the patient or to give his opinion on the quality of medical care at issue in the case. A physician often provides both forms of information. To elicit a witness's testimony, the attorney utilizes one of two available modes. The first and traditional method is the Socratic approach of question and answer, with specific, refined questions and limited, concise answers. The alternative is a narrative format with the attorney asking a relatively broad question that permits the witness to provide an even broader response. Generally, the latter format is more effective since audiences are more attentive to a narrative description than to one that is halting and interrupted by questions. For example, the statement "Please describe for the court your professional training and experience subsequent to high school" generally elicits not only the physician's qualifications more effectively than specific questions about college, medical school, internship, residency, board certification, teaching experience, clinical experience, etc., but also the witness's credibility, conveyed by his demeanor of either modesty or conceit and arrogance. However, some courts insist on a specific question-and-answer format. Communication is extremely important so that both the attorney and the witness are aware of the form of questioning to be employed, since it bears directly on how the witness's trial testimony will be perceived.

Before 1976, regardless of the format chosen, there was only one universally accepted device for eliciting an expert opinion—the hypothetical question. This type of question is rather lengthy and effectively enables the attorney to give a free summary of his case to the jury. In a typical hypothetical question, the attorney recites all the facts in evidence that are relevant to the formation of an opinion; the witness is then asked, assuming the facts recited to be true, whether he is able to form an opinion therefrom and, if so, to state his opinion. In a case involving alleged malpractice in childbirth resulting in cerebral palsy, for example, the question would have to enumerate in detail all of the relevant history and treatment during pregnancy, labor, delivery, and the description of injuries. All of the facts necessary for the witness's opinion will have to be included in the question, and thus, it should be prepared carefully with the attorney prior to trial.

In 1976, the federal courts adopted a new set of evidentiary rules which many of the states have begun adopting in their own courts. One of the most significant changes in the rules of evidence provided for the expression of expert opinions without using a hypothetical question. The modern approach adopted by the federal courts permits an attorney to ask an expert for his opinion by merely asking it without an elaborate preface of factual suppositions.

During direct examination, the witness is asked questions liberally sprinkled with *why* and *how*. Such questions provide the witness with the opportunity to explain or to teach the jury the bases for his opinions. If charts or diagrams are to be used, a small collapsible pointer adds a professional touch to the testimony, especially when an opposing witness merely points at the chart with his finger and blocks the view of the jury by standing in front of the exhibit.

Cross-Examination

At the conclusion of his direct examination, the witness experiences major concern in anticipation of being exposed to the crucible of cross-examination. The scope of cross-examination may be limited to the subject matter brought out during direct examination. However, the cross-examiner avoids repetition of the direct testimony in favor of dwelling on the two principal objectives of cross-examination: establishing those points where he feels he can either provide support for his own case or discredit the witness's testimony.

Much of the earlier discussion regarding depositions is equally appropriate in understanding cross-examination, e.g., the comments regarding learned treatises, repetition of unclear questions, control of temper, and the stare tactic. A cross-examiner uses leading questions as his primary format. His questions are carefully drafted, setting forth a fact or an opinion seeking to get the witness to concur with the fact or opinion suggested in the question. If even the slightest element of the question needs to be clarified, explained, or changed before the witness is able to give a yes or no answer, then the witness must point out his concern before responding to the question. The need to pay careful attention to the propounded question cannot be overemphasized. The leading question is designed to get the witness to agree with the remarks made by the attorney and to provide support for the cross-examiner's theory of the case.

The second principal objective of cross-examination, discrediting the testimony of a witness, can be achieved through one or more of the five following procedures:

1. *Contrary evidence* is nothing more than presenting other witnesses or documentary evidence that is in direct conflict and contradicts the

witness. Cross-examination elicits and solidifies the witness's testimony on the controversial matter.

2. *Bias* can be established with any type of information or disclosure about a witness that might keep him from rendering an impartial opinion, such as a personal prejudice or any emotional, financial, or family relationship with the party for whom he is testifying. Because expert testimony is intended to be an impartial evaluation of the quality of medical care, a defendant-physician should avoid calling one of his partners in practice as an expert witness on his behalf; however, calling a professional acquaintance is ordinarily appropriate.

3. *Character attack* is based upon information challenging a witness's credentials or establishing that the witness's practice is inconsistent with what he is preaching. For those witnesses who are charlatans and who hold themselves out as possessing significant credentials or experience that they in fact do not possess, this tactic provides an exceptional method for impeaching their testimony.

4. *Capacity defect,* the inability of a witness to observe or remember, such as a failure to consider relevant information important to formulating an opinion, can undercut the whole thrust of his opinion. For example, if an anesthesiologist testifies about certain surgical aspects of an operation at which he provided anesthesia, and if it can be pointed out on cross-examination that he could not possibly have observed those aspects of the surgery and that his testimony is thus based upon something other than his own perceptions, his entire testimony would be subject to disbelief.

5. *Prior inconsistent statements,* a device that highlights the significance of discovery depositions, are the most effective and frequently used mode of impeaching or attacking the credibility of witnesses. While a discovery deposition is the primary source of a prior inconsistent statement, alternative sources can be the witness's publications, speeches, or testimony given by the same witness in another lawsuit. When confronted with a prior inconsistent statement on the witness stand, the witness can admit or deny that he made the statement. If he admits it, counsel has scored his point; if the witness denies it, counsel most likely is prepared to prove that the statement was made by producing a witness or a document to support his view, thus successfully impeaching the credibility of the witness. No one is expected to have total recall of every statement they have ever made, and a judge and jury will have little patience with a lawyer who attempts to discredit a witness by bringing up minor, immaterial inconsistencies. Accordingly, a witness's concern about impeachment based upon prior inconsistent state-

ments should not be centered on insignificant inconsistencies normally associated with an individual's ability to recall past events.

Conclusion

Medical malpractice litigation demands the cooperation of both the medical and legal communities. When this goal is achieved, attorneys can then truly represent the interests of the respective parties to the litigation and provide confidence in and acceptance of the adversary system.

Chapter 8

Testifying in Medical-Legal Cases

James G. Zimmerly

Testifying in court is an unavoidable part of medical practice.[1] Actively practicing physicians and surgeons must face the issue with some frequency. It need not be a totally frustrating and unsatisfying role. Physicians can expect to be called to testify in both civil (usually personal injury) and criminal (oftentimes sexual assault) cases. Physicians may find themselves testifying as ordinary factual witnesses or as expert witnesses.

The physician who is called to testify as a factual witness is limited in his testimony to facts within his personal knowledge, and he is not permitted to render an opinion.[2] The factual witness testifies to what he saw and what he did. A couple of examples of factual testimony are "I saw the 1949 Chevy go through the red light at First and Main Street at noon on December 24" and "I treated Mrs. Jones for a spontaneous abortion on December 24 in the emergency room of Memorial Hospital." If the physician recorded in the patient's medical record that Mrs. Jones was hit by a 1949 Chevy that ran a red light at First and Main Street, that portion of the medical record would not be admissible because the physician was not an actual witness to the accident.[3] Mrs. Jones may have told the physician that information during his collection of a medical history, but the physician cannot testify to it. There are two exceptions:

1. the judge may allow or sometimes order such testimony; and
2. it may be admissable as an exception to the hearsay rule in some courts.

Expert witnesses not only may testify to the facts within their personal knowledge, but may also give opinions based on the facts and based on hypothetical questions. Hypothetical questions must conform to the facts in evidence in the case.[4] An exchange based on a brief hypothetical question* might be as follows:

Attorney: Assume that Mrs. Jones was sitting motionless in her car when she was hit from behind by a car traveling less than twenty-five miles per hour. Assume that Mrs. Jones developed vaginal bleeding twelve hours after the accident and spontaneously aborted. Doctor, do you have an opinion, based on reasonable medical certainty, whether Mrs. Jones's abortion was caused by the rear end accident?

Physician: Yes, I have an opinion.

Attorney: What is that opinion?

Physician: [At this point the physician states his opinion.]

The testimony of the expert is grounded in the education, training, skill, and experience of that individual. The same is true of an expert in any field, whether it be medical practice, ballistics, toxicology, or any other scientific field. Expert testimony is not required if the matter under review is within the common knowledge of judges and/or juries.† For instance, expert testimony is not required to advise the court that an x-ray should have been taken when a serious fracture was suspected.

Before the Trial

Subpoena

A subpoena is a court order demanding that an individual "appear at a certain time and place to give testimony upon a certain matter"

---

* Hypothetical questions are usually not so abbreviated; many more facts would be necessary if the question were asked during an actual proceeding.

† In some situations, expert testimony may not be required. The court may take judicial notice of certain facts, but these are generally limited to extraordinarily common knowledge. The trial judge makes this decision. Usually, a trial attorney attempts to establish his case by expert testimony, even those elements that would seem to be apparent even to the most unsophisticated juror. See Chapter 9, Putting Res Ipsa Loquitur and Informed Consent in Perspective, for a more detailed explanation.

(p. 1279).[5] Receiving a subpoena may be the physician's first indication that he is being called to testify as a factual witness in a case. A subpoena should not be ignored. Some physicians have done so and have been fined for contempt of court.[6,7] Usually the physician who treated the plaintiff-patient will be subpoenaed and must testify as a factual witness, and in some states he may be asked expert witness questions. On the other hand, a physician who did not treat the plaintiff-patient cannot be called to testify as an expert witness unless he agrees to do so in advance of the trial. However, if an expert witness agrees to testify for the plaintiff-patient and then, for whatever reason, decides to back out and if the patient loses the case, the expert witness may become a defendant in a breach of contract action.

Deposition

The deposition, in some instances, may save a trip to the courtroom.[8] The purpose of the deposition is discovery of all the facts for all parties to the litigation. It is less formal and is usually conducted in one of the lawyer's offices. Despite the informality, the witness is under oath and whatever is stated in the deposition may be used to impeach his credibility should he later change his story during the trial. In fact, before testifying at the trial, the witness should read his deposition in preparation for his appearance in court.

The witness should prepare for the deposition just as he would for courtroom testimony. Cavalier comments should not be made just because the setting is relaxed and informal; these statements may be read back during the trial to embarrass the witness. Attorneys may raise objections during the deposition that are directed at both the form and the substance of the questions that are asked. If the attorney representing the side that has sought the witness's testimony objects to the form of the opposing attorney's questions, then the question must be rephrased. If the attorney objects to the substance of the question and queries whether it would be admissible in court, the objection is made and stated in the record, but then the witness must proceed to answer the question. At a later date, arguments will be held to determine whether the question will be admissible during the trial.

Preparation

The expert witness should obtain and review all records and materials pertinent to the case. The expert should intensely study the subject, but should not attempt to memorize his testimony. The expert should be prepared to explain the reasons for differing medical opinions or differing types of treatment for the same condition. The expert should be certain that the facts support the medical theory upon which he is testifying. He should then correlate these facts with the temporal sequence of events.

The expert should insist on a pretrial conference with the attorney who has called him.[9] The attorney should prepare the expert for direct examination as well as for cross-examination. A good direct examination will often neutralize the cross-examination. If the cross-examining attorney asks the expert witness if he discussed the case with the other attorney, the answer would be "Yes, we discussed the subject matter involved in this case as well as how to present it to the jury clearly and effectively."

The expert should be familiar with his own curriculum vitae, although it need not be memorized. Credentials should be neither exaggerated nor played down. The expert and the attorney who is calling him should agree in advance on those parts of the curriculum vitae that will be brought out to establish the expert's qualifications.

The expert should be informed about where to go and where to wait at the courthouse. He should enter the courtroom only as arranged with the attorney. Spontaneously walking into the courtroom could result in a mistrial in certain courts where experts are prohibited from listening to other witnesses' testimony. A further, practical suggestion is that the expert witness should have an empty bladder before going on the stand. He has no control over how long he will be sitting on the stand.

Fee

The fee to be received by a witness should be set in advance. The basic fee for testifying as a factual witness may be a standard amount.* An expert witness, on the other hand, can set his own fee based on the time he spends in preparing his testimony, in giving a deposition, in presenting his courtroom testimony, and even in traveling to and from the courthouse.

The witness should not make an issue of the fee in the courtroom. For example, there are a few states where factual witnesses, such as

---

* The standard fee for factual witnesses is usually reimbursement for mileage or no fee at all.

treating physicians, can be forced to answer expert witness questions. The witness who argues with the judge that his professional opinion is a property right which he cannot be forced to give away free of charge may go directly to jail.

How do expert witnesses set their fees? Some physicians charge a lump sum for their entire involvement with a case. The problem with this arrangement is that a $2,000 lump sum may at first sound outrageously high, but, in fact, it may not be adequate compensation for the time spent on the case. Other physicians set an hourly rate. The expert should not agree to work on a contingent fee basis; not only will it ruin his credibility with the jury, but it is unethical. The witness can expect to be asked during the trial how much he is being paid for his testimony. The witness should reply, "I am not being paid for my testimony. I do expect to be paid for my time, my professional knowledge, my services in studying the facts of this case, and for my opinion based on those facts." If the witness is asked how much his fee is, an hourly sum appears to be more modest and tasteful than a flat fee of several thousand dollars.

The expert should prepare a bill for both the attorney and the client, unless the attorney agrees in advance to be responsible for the fee. The agreement should entitle the expert to be paid for his services if the case is settled. The agreement should not be based only on time spent testifying in court, since most cases never get to the courtroom. If the lawyer does not pay the fee, the witness should report him to his local bar association before considering bringing suit against him. The grievance committee of the local bar association will review the case, and if they agree with the expert's position, they will force the attorney to pay the fee.

In the Courtroom

Direct Examination

Since an expert witness is permitted not only to testify about the facts in a case but also to express opinions and conclusions drawn from those facts, it must be demonstrated before his testimony is given that the witness is qualified to testify as an expert. Qualifying the expert requires a great deal of preparation by the examining attorney. The questions that will be asked to establish the witness's expertise must be planned in advance and tailored to that individual expert. An expert witness whose credentials are impressive should be permitted to state his qualifications in response to specific questions so that the jury has an opportunity to be favorably impressed. Opposing counsel might offer to stipulate the expertise of the witness under the guise of saving the court's time, when in fact the real reason is to minimize the consideration that the jury might attribute to such imposing qualifications.[2,10]

The direct examination of a witness should be planned and rehearsed well in advance of the trial so that it is a relaxed experience.[11] The expert should not answer the question before it is asked. He should take his time and listen carefully. He should not volunteer information on either direct or cross-examination. He should be specific, brief, and to the point.[12] The expert appears unsure of himself if he constantly hedges when answering questions by using "I suppose" or "it appears" or "indications are." He should act like a surgeon rather than an internist. He should not try to lead or to help the lawyer. The witness should retain his professional objectivity at all times.

Cross-Examination

The cross-examination of witnesses is considered a safeguard of accuracy and an indispensable technique for the discovery of truth.[13] Cross-examination has three main functions:

1. to shed light on the credibility of the direct testimony;
2. to bring out additional facts related to those elicited during direct examination; and
3. in states following the wide open rule,* to bring out additional facts that might elucidate any issue in the case.

After a witness has been questioned in direct examination, the other party has the right to cross-examine that witness to ascertain and exhibit the situation of the witness with respect to the parties and to the subject of litigation—his interests, his motives, his inclinations, his prejudices, his means of obtaining a correct and certain knowledge of the facts to which he has borne testimony, the manner in which he has used those means, and his powers of discernment, memory, and description. The purposes of the cross-examination are to test the truthfulness of the witness, to sift, modify, or explain what has been said, to develop new

---

* The court that adopts the "wide open rule" permits the cross-examination to be almost unlimited, i.e., not limited to what is asked on direct examination.

or old facts in a view favorable to the cross-examiner, or to discredit the witness.

The right of cross-examination is absolute and is not a mere privilege of the one against whom a witness may be called. If a party, through no fault of his own, has been deprived of an opportunity to cross-examine an opposing witness, he would be permitted to have the direct evidence stricken from the record. A party who puts a friendly witness on the witness stand is not permitted to cross-examine that witness except where it can be shown to the satisfaction of the court:

1. that the testimony of the witness is a surprise to the party calling him;
2. that it is inconsistent with other statements made by the witness; or
3. that the witness is hostile.

The witness must expect to be vigorously cross-examined about his qualifications as well as his scientific findings and even his character. The expert's knowledge and experience will be tested by questions before he is permitted to testify on the facts of the case; these questions will be directed at the witness's competency. The expert witness should not be drawn into a feeling of antagonism merely because the cross-examiner expresses a doubtful attitude about the expert's opinion. The expert witness whose credentials are slim may be permitted to testify if the judge feels that he meets the minimum requirements for expert testimony on the facts at issue. However, minimal credentials could result in the testimony receiving less weight or credibility than that given by a more prominent, experienced expert. During cross-examination, the expert's minimal experience will be emphasized by the attorney in order to convince the jury to give low weight to this expert's opinion.[10]

The expert witness must realize that the cross-examining attorney will attempt to discredit him as well as his testimony. This unpleasant, personal attack is sometimes difficult for the expert, but it can be tolerated once the witness understands and accepts the fact that he is functioning within an adversary system. By description, this system is a contest of unfriendly opponents. The judge, however, can protect the witness during cross-examination from questions that are merely intended to harass, annoy, or humiliate. It is inappropriate for the attorney, without foundation in the evidence, to question the integrity and veracity of respectable witnesses by suggesting that they are liars or that they have been or could have been bought.

The widest range of questioning that is permitted during cross-examination occurs when a witness is impeached.[14] The purpose of impeaching an adverse witness is to impair his credibility by showing that there are contradictions in his statements, that his reputation for telling the truth is bad, that the facts are other than he states them to be, or that he is biased about the case.

While cross-examination puts the witness in the hot seat, the witness can survive and can handle the tactics used by even the greatest of lawyers. Here are some guidelines for the witness who wants to retain his integrity and credibility as an expert under the most grueling cross-examination. The witness should always remain calm and remain polite to the cross-examining attorney; that will undo the attorney and not the witness. The witness should not allow himself to be lulled into a false sense of security by a "good humor" lawyer. The witness should ignore all the officious paper shuffling and writing that the cross-examining attorney may do. The witness should not change his demeanor or his tone as he goes from direct examination to cross-examination.

The witness must be alert and think, think, think at all times to avoid carefully laid traps. For example, here is a typical exchange in the cross-examination of a treating physician who is called as a witness.

Attorney: Are you a friend of the patient?

Physician: I try to be a friend to all of my patients.

Attorney: Would you not like to see your friend win this case?

Physician: I am here to give impartial medical testimony and not to decide the case. I am sure the jury will do a good job of that.

The expert witness should not become caught in a tempo of answering short, rapid-fire questions calling for "yes" answers, because a question calling for a "no" answer may be slipped in. The expert should not anticipate. Neither should he relax once he thinks the questioning is over; he should wait until he hears the magic words "That is all, doctor."

If the witness appears frequently as a medical expert witness, he should be prepared to answer questions about his propensity to spend time in court. If he is an out-of-town expert, he should be prepared to state why he traveled so far to testify in this case. One compelling reason may well be that his qualifications are especially well suited to the issues in the case. If the cross-examination drags on interminably, he should remain calm because he is probably ahead on points with the jury, and the cross-examining attorney is desperately trying to break him down. The witness should pass up the opportunity to "zing" the cross-examining attorney. More cross-examinations are suicidal than they are homicidal. The cross-examining attorney should be fair to the witness, lest he run the risk of increasing the sympathy that the jury feels toward the witness and increasing the antagonism that they feel toward the lawyer. If the cross-examination is nothing more than a repetition of the questions that were asked of the witness on direct examination, the effect will be to reinforce the expert's answers. If the jury hears the same question answered the same way over and over, that testimony may be the only one they recall during their later deliberations.[14]

If the attorney intends to rely on a medical treatise or textbook to cross-examine the expert witness, the witness must establish the treatise as authoritative or the text will not be admitted into evidence.[13] However, the federal rules of evidence do permit the court to conclude that certain texts are authoritative and to permit their use.[15] Some experts attempt to avoid cross-examination on a particular text by stating that their opinion is based on their own experience and observation, as well as on the reading of many books and journal articles about the subject and not on one particular treatise. There are a growing number of cases in which the courts have permitted treatises or technical books to be used in the cross-examination of an expert witness in order to test the witness's competency or qualifications regardless of whether the witness relied upon or recognized the authoritative status of the treatise.[16]

Guidelines for a Court Appearance

Besides the witness's actual verbal testimony, many other factors influence the jury's perception of his credibility, such as his dress, comfort, and attitude.* The witness should be on time to give his testimony and should not talk to others about the case while waiting to be called. He should dress comfortably and not too flashy; he should not wear lapel buttons. Once on the stand, the witness should sit up straight or lean forward a bit to better hear the questions, clasp his hands lightly, and plant both feet on the floor. The witness should look at the jurors when giving an answer and should use language that they

---

* See Chapter 10, Nonverbal Communication in the Courtroom, for a detailed discussion.

can understand. The witness who cannot communicate effectively with the jury cannot help to win the case for the side that called him.

The medical witness should concentrate on always being courteous to the judge, the jury, and the lawyers.[2] The expert should be professional in his remarks but should not be pompous or talk down to the judge and jury. A condescending or smug attitude will not favorably impress the jury, while an attitude of modesty may very well have a strong impact. It is never appropriate to argue with the judge.

If possible, the witness should use charts or models to explain the case to the jury. Jurors are impressed by evidence that they can see. Photographs and x-rays may be helpful. Color photographs are better than black and white, and models that contain moving parts are most influential.

The medical expert witness should remain calm while under even the most vigorous cross-examination. The confident, prepared, and truthful expert witness cannot be embarrassed or unsettled by even the best lawyer's questions. The cross-examiner who is unable to discredit the testimony of the witness may resort to methods calculated to irritate the physician in an attempt to cause him to lose his temper. The witness gains nothing by overreacting to this type of behavior by the attorney. It is a deliberate trap set to shake up the witness. If it fails by the witness retaining his composure, the witness will gain a valuable plus with the jurors in their assessment of his entire appearance on the witness stand.[17]

While the role of an expert witness in any case is not likely to become the favorite pastime of more than a few unusual physicians, it need not be a demeaning or unpleasant experience if the witness is prepared, relaxed, and truthful.

Summary:
Dos and Don'ts for the Witness[18,19]

Dos

- Do appear professional, relaxed, and calm.
- Do answer only the questions asked.
- Do speak clearly and confidently.
- Do use understandable language.
- Do speak directly to the jury.
- Do be yourself.

Don'ts

- Don't volunteer information.
- Don't answer if you don't understand the question.
- Don't hesitate to say "I don't know."
- Don't argue with the judge or the attorneys.
- Don't underestimate the attorneys.
- Don't challenge the attorneys in their forum.
- Don't talk down to the jury.
- Don't try to act out a role.

References

1. Strodel, RC. Medical legal relationships: a physician's patient is the same person as an attorney's client. Leg Aspects Med Pract 6(3):54, 1978.
2. Zimmerly, JG. Clinical forensic medicine. *In* Forensic sciences, CH Wecht, ed, pp 221–235. New York: Matthew Bender, 1981.
3. Hirsch, CS, Morris, RC, and Moritz, AR. Handbook of legal medicine, ed 5. St Louis: CV Mosby, 1979.
4. 31 Am Jur 2d, Expert and Opinion Evidence, §56, 1967.
5. Black, HC. Black's law dictionary, ed 5. St Paul, MN: West Publishing Co, 1979.
6. *People v. Florendo,* 95 Ill 2d 155; 447 NE2d 282, 1983.
7. *People v. Herbert,* 438 NE2d 1255, 1982.
8. Jowers, LV. It's your job. J Leg Med 5(4):8u, 1977.
9. Lewin, HW. The medical legal examination and testimony—an ophthalmologist's view. J Leg Med 3(3):35, 1975.
10. Exter, FB, Jr. How to be an expert witness. J Leg Med 4(10):17, 1976.
11. Selecting and preparing expert witnesses. 2 Am Jur Trials 585, 1964.
12. Waltz, JR and Inbau, FE. Medical jurisprudence. New York: Macmillan, 1971.
13. Curran, WJ and Shapiro, DE. Law, medicine and forensic science. Boston: Little, Brown, 1970.
14. Moenssens, AA and Inbau, FE. Scientific evidence in criminal cases. Mineola, NY: The Foundation Press, 1978.
15. Fed R Evid 803(18).
16. Use of medical or other scientific treatises in cross-examination of expert witnesses. 60 ALR2d 77.
17. Reed, JW. Cross examination of the medical expert, personal injury and technique (Source handbook series, vol 4). New York: Practicing Law Institute, 1968.
18. Horsley, JE and Carlova, J. Testifying in court: a guide for physicians, ed 2. Oradell, NJ: Medical Economics Books, 1983.
19. Curran, WJ. Tracy's the doctor as a witness, ed 2. Philadelphia: WB Saunders, 1965.

Chapter 9

Putting Res Ipsa Loquitur and Informed Consent in Perspective

Jeffrey A. Shane

In both the legal and medical literature on medical malpractice, two topics have received more than their fair share of attention—res ipsa loquitur and informed consent. Most of this attention is substantially greater than is actually warranted, promoting unreasonable anticipation and fear within the medical community. Addressing these topics directly will help medical practitioners put these two legal doctrines into an appropriately balanced perspective.

Res Ipsa Loquitur

Res ipsa loquitur, which literally means "the thing speaks for itself," is a doctrine invoked in cases of obvious negligence. The keystone case in the application of this doctrine was *Ybarra v. Spangard,* decided by the Supreme Court of California in 1944.[1] After undergoing an appendectomy, the patient awoke with weakness in his arm, which subsequently developed into paresis and atrophy of the shoulder girdle muscles. The patient brought suit against the operating surgeon, the hospital owner, the anesthetist, and at least one of the nurses. The defendants in the case argued that it was unclear how this injury occurred, and since it would be impossible to determine who might be at fault, none of them should be held liable. The court, in finding for the plaintiff, applied the doctrine of res ipsa loquitur, pointing out that without this doctrine the legal maxim "for every wrong, there is a remedy" could not be applied. The court stated that without the aid of this doctrine

> a patient who received permanent injuries of a serious character, obviously the result of someone's negligence, would be entirely unable to recover unless the doctors and nurses in attendance voluntarily chose to disclose the identity of the negligent person and the facts establishing liability.

In what has become known as the *Ybarra* rule, the court identified three conditions for applying the doctrine of res ipsa loquitur. First, the injury-causing accident must be one that ordinarily does not occur unless someone is negligent. Second, the injury must be caused by an agency or instrumentality that is in the exclusive control of the defendants. Third, there must be no contributory action by the injured plaintiff. The court felt that previous decisions in the state of California supported the view that when a plaintiff's injuries are so clearly the result of someone's negligence, the defendant is required to explain the unusual result:

> where a plaintiff receives unusual injuries while unconscious and in the course of medical treatment, all those defendants who had any control over his body or the instrumentality which might have caused the injury, may properly be called upon to meet the inference of negligence by giving an explanation of their conduct.

Even though this doctrine has received fairly wide application and has not been confined exclusively to the medical malpractice arena, the results of another California malpractice case, *Folk v. Kilk,* define the limits of the doctrine of res ipsa loquitur.[2] In this case, a malpractice action was brought against an ear, nose, and throat specialist by a patient who developed a brain abscess shortly after having a tonsillectomy. The court pointed out that in malpractice cases arising from surgical procedures, the second and third elements of the *Ybarra* rule are usually inherent, i.e., the patient is usually under the exclusive control of the doctor and/or hospital and generally performs no voluntary action that might contribute to his injury. The court, therefore, focused upon the first element of the *Ybarra* rule—the accident must be one that ordinarily does not occur in the absence of someone's negligence. Since the etiology of brain abscess and standard of care concerning tonsillectomies are not matters of common knowledge, the court was bound by expert testimony that would establish whether or not the injury resulted from negligence. In other words, the court restricted the doctrine of res ipsa loquitur to those cases in which even the most unsophisticated individual in medical matters would conclude that the injury occurred because someone was negligent. For example, the doctrine may be applied in cases where foreign bodies are left in patients, especially when no emergency situation required the rapid cessation of the operative procedure. Another example is the patient whose injury is far distant from the site of the operation, is totally unrelated to the operative procedure, and is, therefore, almost certainly the result of an accident that occurred during the surgery.

The doctrine is rarely applied to an injury that is directly associated with the surgical procedure itself. Therefore, in cases where unfortunate intraoperative outcomes are directly related to the procedure itself, the burden of proof will be on the plaintiff, who will have to produce expert testimony that violation of an appropriate standard of care resulted in this injury.

The important lesson for the practicing physician is that the threat of a lawsuit based on this doctrine can often be eliminated by good risk management within the medical care facility. Careful survey of operative suites and rigid adherence to safety protocols will eliminate the majority of such injuries and decrease to near zero the situations in which this doctrine can be applied. Res ipsa loquitur is not a doctrine to be ignored; rather, it should be a reminder that risk management procedures can significantly decrease the incidence of malpractice actions.

Informed Consent

The legal doctrine of informed consent has undergone major revisions in the last three decades, spawning controversy and confusion. The court decisions that brought about these revisions were influenced by several factors:

> [1] the courts' perspective is necessarily shaped by their near-exclusive experience with injured, unhappy patients . . . . [2] courts see only those cases in which particular allegedly undisclosed risks associated with medical procedures have led to actual injuries . . . . [3] courts must grapple with difficulties posed by the impact of hindsight on the litigation process . . . . [4] courts must determine whether required disclosures were in fact made . . . . Taken together, these have brought the current law to an uneasy compromise among ethical aspirations, the realities of medical practice, and the exigencies of the litigation process [pp. 25–29].[3]

The uncertainty surrounding the law's requirements and the physician's accountability during this time of flux has created concern that is out of proportion with the doctrine's legal presence. To develop a more appropriate, balanced perspective of informed consent, the physician needs to begin with an understanding of the doctrine's foundations in tort law.* This introduction leads to an exploration of what information the patient requires, how accountability is determined, and what exceptions can be invoked. The controversy surrounding the informed consent doctrine is rooted in the confusing answers the law has given to these questions. Answering these questions

> is clearly no simple task, either for the law that must formulate disclosure standards or for practitioners who must apply those standards to the myriad individual circumstances that arise in medical practice. Nor is the conflict ... unique to the law of informed consent. Indeed, this conflict represents an important limitation on the law as an instrument of social control [p. 72].[3]

Battery†

In both civil and criminal cases, the term *battery* refers to any intentional, unconsented touching of another. In order to bring an action in battery, the claimant needs only to show that the unconsented touching did, in fact, occur to establish a prima facie case.

> [The] law does not require the patient to be physically damaged by the intervention. His health may be significantly improved, and yet the doctor is liable. Nor is proof required that the patient's probable conduct in submitting to the touching would have been different, had the doctor fulfilled his duty to disclose the nature of the procedure. In some of the cases, the plaintiff, knowing what was intended, would very likely have agreed. Thus, a successful battery action may provide the plaintiff with free care, improved health, and financial compensation. The arguable inequity of this result is

---

* See Chapter 4, The Historic Basis of Medical-Legal Liability, for a detailed discussion.

† Doctrines of consent and informed consent are included under the general topic of battery since they arose from early actions on this tort. There has certainly been substantial intermingling of the traditional battery action and the more current actions for negligence or lack of informed consent. However, the common practice in most courts is to consider actions for lack of informed consent as negligence actions rather than as actions for intentional tort such as battery. This practice is perhaps based on the notion that "the withholding of information on the part of physicians is generally quite intentional, dictated by the very exercise of medical judgment which the law of negligence, unlike the law of battery, seeks to respect" (p. 166).[4]

overridden by the great fear that something will be done to a person which
he did not invite and had no opportunity to veto, however medically appropriate it may be [p. 145].[4]

However, under a wide variety of circumstances, the individual im-
plicitly consents to certain touchings. For example, a commuter who
rides the subway in a large city during rush hour has given implied
consent to a moderate amount of jostling and crowding; the passenger
who is "touched" in the press of the crowd is unlikely to be successful
in a battery action. The person who enters a medical treatment facility
gives a certain implied consent to medical treatment. Unless written
consent is required by statute or other regulation, consent to any form
of touching may be verbal. For many treatment modalities, it may be
implied by the very presence of the patient within the treatment facility.
In response to rising malpractice litigation and the need to document
this consent in case of a future contest, many health care facilities have
constructed formal, written consent forms.

In an emergency situation, the patient's consent is implied. A common example is the injured patient who is found unconscious and
brought to a treatment facility where he receives emergency lifesaving
treatment. Courts have generally held that under such circumstances
the health care provider may assume the individual would have requested and consented to medical treatment that would save life or
limb. Such implied consent applies to virtually any procedure that
would preserve life and limb and continues until the individual is able
to make a rational decision to continue or reject further treatment.

Under the reverse circumstances, however, the court is not quite as
lenient. Specifically, if the patient who begins the course of treatment
is competent, conscious, of proper age, and otherwise able to give
consent but is later rendered unconscious, as for example by anesthesia,
the health care provider cannot assume that the individual would have
consented to procedures beyond the scope originally contemplated,
unless a truly life-threatening, immediate situation occurs. No health
care provider would allow a patient to die or sustain serious injury
purely because no consent had been obtained. On the other hand,
elective or semielective procedures, even though cost effective and easily
performed in one sitting, must be deferred pending consultation with
the patient, unless the matter was discussed ahead of time. For these
reasons, the courts have found it reasonable for the health care provider
to discuss with the patient the reasonable risks and alternatives to any
proposed treatment, including such things as other procedures that
might be required at the same time. This compendium of the risks,

alternatives, and potential complications of any mode of medical treatment constitutes what most jurisdictions generally require for a patient's consent to be considered informed.

Sometimes a fine line exists between the indicated operative procedure and what might be considered beyond the scope of the original operation. For example, in the case of *Mohr v. Williams,* the patient had gone to the physician for problems with her right ear.[5] After the anesthetic was administered, the physician concluded that the malady affecting the right ear was not serious enough to require surgery; however, he determined that the left ear did, indeed, need surgical correction. The operation was successfully performed. The patient brought an action in battery, and the trial court found for the plaintiff in the amount of $14,322.50. On appeal, the Minnesota Supreme Court pointed out that a physician must not be prevented from taking measures in a case he considers to be an emergency; however, in this case, the act of the defendant amounted to technical battery. The court noted that any unauthorized touching, except in the spirit of pleasantry, constitutes assault and battery and, being unauthorized, is unlawful; but unlike a criminal prosecution, there is no need for unlawful intent. The court concluded that the amount of the recovery should depend upon the character and extent of the injury inflicted upon the patient and that the good faith of the defendant should be taken into consideration. At a second trial, the plaintiff received a verdict in her favor with a judgment for $39.00. Although such an outcome appears to be an almost total vindication of the physician, he was forced to endure the trauma and loss of time entailed in going through two trials. Further, had he chosen not to appeal the original trial verdict, he would have been liable for the total amount of the judgment as entered by the trial level court.

What Information Does the Patient Require?

The recurrent question faced by the practitioner is just how much information the patient needs to be given. While some have suggested that the patient requires an extensive medical education, others have proposed extensive informed consent documents that list every potential complication of every procedure from phlebitis at the site of an intravenous portal to grotesque and horrible death. Conceivably, if a patient suffers even a very minor and very rare adverse outcome about which she was not specifically informed, some court, somewhere, might find liability due to lack of informed consent. Although there is no way to guard against such nitpicking, most jurisdictions will not go to such extremes. Instead, some courts look at what a reasonable patient in the same or similar circumstances as the patient would expect to be told about the procedure and its risks; other jurisdictions may hold the standard to be that which the reasonable physician would tell a patient in the same or similar circumstances. Generally, the more elective the procedure, the higher the standard to which a court will hold the physician in informing the patient of the potential risks. Thus, a patient faced with an urgent and serious medical situation would likely not prevail in an action for failure to disclose a minor or insignificant risk. On the other end of the spectrum, the patient undergoing a totally cosmetic, elective operative procedure has a right to thorough counseling regarding the possible risks of this proposed operation.

To outline for any and every operative procedure exactly what the patient must be told is impossible. Most courts hold that the physician should certainly inform the patient of the more serious complications and the likelihood of their occurrence. Such things as death, prolonged hospitalization, loss of limb function, significant scarring, or prolonged pain would be things that any reasonable patient would expect to know before undergoing an operative procedure. In addition, the hazards related to specific operative procedures are included in this category. For example, a patient undergoing a sterilization procedure is specifically looking forward to no further pregnancies. It is, therefore, incumbent upon the treating physician to counsel the patient about the risk of pregnancy following such a procedure, as well as the various alternative modes of sterilization and contraception, the risks associated with each, and specifically the risk of pregnancy following each.

The physician should begin by appropriately examining and counseling the patient, making it clear what operation is intended, and explaining what modifications may be undertaken should different findings than anticipated actually be noted. For example, the gynecologist who undertakes a surgical exploration of an acute abdomen, where the suspicion is possible ectopic pregnancy or other intraabdominal catastrophe, may find that the cause of the problem is nongynecologic, such as appendicitis or other acute bowel problem. The patient may then be better prepared should she learn that a second surgeon was requested or should she awaken with a colostomy or a bowel resection. Further, when the original operative procedure is intended to investigate an uncertain diagnosis, such as ectopic pregnancy or ruptured cyst, the patient should be cautioned that more extensive surgery may be required. Particularly relevant is the case of the young patient for whom the surgical findings necessitate a hysterectomy. The hysterectomy is no less necessary just because the patient was not informed of this risk; but because of the shock and dismay at having had such a procedure, the patient will be tempted to seek legal counsel. The concern is not with whether the case is defensible, but rather with a way of avoiding litigation in the first place. If these different risks are clearly explained to the patient prior to surgery, the patient is substantially less motivated to consider legal action.

There is an element known in the law as the thin skull doctrine that has not been eliminated. This doctrine was first elucidated in 1901 in the English case of *Dulieu v. White* and exemplified in the influential New York Court of Appeals opinion of *McCahill v. New York Transportation Company*.[6,7] The New York court recognized that

> a negligent person is responsible for the direct effect of his acts, even if more serious, in case of the sick and infirmed as well as in those of healthy and robust people .... [One who] has negligently forwarded a diseased condition, and by that hastened and prematurely caused death, cannot escape responsibility even though the disease probably would have resulted in death at a later time without his agency.

Put into the simplest terms, an ordinary patient requires certain information to be adequately informed of the risks of a procedure; however, a patient who has certain underlying conditions or special circumstances that make her more susceptible to complications needs more individualized information. Thus, it is absolutely impossible to formulate any blanket consent or informed consent document that will cover any operative procedure; rather, every informed consent must be tailored to the individual's needs and underlying state of health. Therefore, in addition to the prospective, reasonable person approach, the court adopted the notion that the reasonable person is in the same or similar circumstances as the particular patient.

The bottom line is that the physician has a duty to ascertain the patient's physical and psychological status as well as to outline the proposed procedure, its goals, and the complications that might be expected to occur with reasonable frequency or which may be serious even if rare. The more serious the complication, the more it needs to be discussed, even if its frequency is somewhat less common. Further, the patient needs to know the reasonable alternatives to the proposed mode of treatment and the risks that these carry. Finally, of course, the patient must be competent to consent to having such a procedure done. This information should be clearly documented in the progress notes or other hospital record and, if possible, in the patient's office record. In addition, a contemporaneously signed operative consent permit is of value and often is required. This permit should indicate that the procedure has been explained to the patient in fairly comprehensible layman's terms and should provide a place for the patient to sign and date it. The document, wherever possible, should be witnessed, preferably by some fairly impartial observer such as a nurse or other member of the health care team who will not be directly involved in the surgical procedure itself.

What Exceptions Can Be Invoked?

All jurisdictions recognize that under certain circumstances disclosure is unnecessary. Following is a brief summary of exceptions which some courts have recognized:

- the patient has foreknowledge of the hazard—the risk is commonly known to the general public and the patient is already aware of the risk;
- the patient voluntarily waives her right to be told of the risk or a reasonable person would have agreed to the treatment whether or not she knew of a particular risk;
- the hazard does not lie within and is not a reasonably foreseeable result of a properly performed, appropriate procedure;
- complete disclosure of the hazards involved would be harmful to the best interests of the patient—therapeutic privilege; or
- an emergency necessitates intervention to prevent death or permanent injury.[8]

Somewhat akin to informed consent are the laws associated with emergency medical care, known in many jurisdictions as Good Samaritan laws. Based loosely on the biblical allegory involving the Good Samaritan, statutory provisions providing limited liability to medical practitioners who in good faith render medical care to a patient under emergency circumstances have been enacted in most jurisdictions. Two basic tenets of virtually all Good Samaritan legislation are that the care rendered must be totally under emergency circumstances and rendered gratuitously. Thus, the health care provider who elects to bill for the services rendered takes the physician-patient relationship outside of the Good Samaritan protection and makes himself liable for any negligence that may have occurred. The laws generally protect the physician until the patient is transported to a facility where sufficient medical care can be rendered or until the patient's care is taken over by another competent health care provider. The liability protection provided is limited to acts of ordinary negligence and would not immunize the health care provider from gross, wanton, or willful acts of negligence. This provision does not apply to a patient who is already under a physician's care and who, because of prior treatment, is placed in an emergency situation that requires remedy. Its original legislative intent was to provide protection for the physician who comes upon an individual who requires immediate care intended to preserve life or limb. A typical example is the physician who witnesses an automobile accident and stops to render assistance.

The broadest interpretation of a Good Samaritan law was made by a California court. This case involved a hospital-based physician who rendered care to a hospitalized patient, not his own, who was in an extremely precarious condition and to whom the physician rendered emergency care. In this particular case, the California court elected to extend the Good Samaritan law to provide liability immunization for this physician.

How Is Accountability Determined?

In *Sard v. Hardy,* the Maryland Court of Appeals analyzed a failed sterilization case in terms of the informed consent issue.[9] The physician selected the Madlener sterilization technique for a postcesarean-section tubal ligation. Although the technique itself was apparently, or at least for purposes of argument, properly performed, the court analyzed the case using the informed consent doctrine. The court reasoned that, given the potential types of sterilization procedures available and the failure rates associated with each of these, a reasonable patient knowing the higher risk of pregnancy with this particular operative procedure might have selected another form of sterilization.

Except in most unusual circumstances, the patient is not allowed a retrospective decision about whether they would have selected a different mode of treatment. Rather, the court may apply the reasonable person standard—given the risks and alternatives, what would a reasonable person have elected—or the reasonable physician standard–what is customarily disclosed? After the fact and with a bad result, almost any patient could honestly allege that knowing the outcome, they would not have selected that particular procedure. Usually, however, the courts apply a prospective approach and look at the modality that a reasonable patient might have elected to undergo before the course of therapy.

Deserving of further discussion are those procedures considered novel or experimental. These procedures range from one extreme, the well-planned, clinically controlled, single-, double-, or even triple-blind experimental protocol, to the other, the procedure devised by the individual physician that has no support from any reasonable segment of the practicing community. The wide acceptance of a medical procedure or rationale of therapy reduces the likelihood of physician liability, but does not guarantee defensibility. In a trial, the defendant-physician is often held to the condition that he

> exercise such reasonable care and skill . . . as is usually exercised by physicians or surgeons in good standing, of the same system or school of practice in the community in which he resides, having due regard to the condition of medical or surgical science at that time.[10]

Included in this category could be the practice of prescribing drugs for indications other than those listed in the package inserts or the Physician's Desk Reference (PDR) without informing the patient about the unconventional usage. "Prescribing for an unlabeled indication does not in itself constitute malpractice, but the package insert along with medical articles, texts, and expert opinion constitutes evidence of proper prescribing."[11] While some suggest that patient package inserts should include a clause stating that the drug may have therapeutic indications other than those specifically listed, the most defensible position is to inform the patient of such usage, to involve the patient in the decision to use it, and to document the patient's informed consent and the physician's rationale in the medical record. Not only will it save scrambling through the literature later to prove what the standard of care was at the time the incident occurred, but it also reflects the physician's due care and consideration which greatly aids in the defensibility of a malpractice action. In addition, should the treatment modality indeed prove to be detrimental or ineffective, the considerations given at the time of its usage become extremely critical.

Summary

Although the doctrine is widely discussed and debated, few cases have been decided solely on the issue of informed consent. Generally, it is included in a list of many other allegations. The confusion surrounding this complicated legal and ethical question has been met with negativism by the medical profession. While an ethical discussion is not within the scope of this chapter, "the broader context of relations

and communications between patients and health care professionals"
(p. 1) must be addressed before the controversy can be resolved.[3]

Listed in Table 1 are guidelines for dealing with informed consent
in the daily practice of medicine. These guidelines again emphasize the
importance of risk management procedures in providing protection in
case of a future action. Critics of defensive medicine may say that the
physician, in an attempt to avoid liability, ends up treating the chart
instead of the patient. The competent physician's response should be
that before establishing a treatment plan, he considers all of the factors
of the patient's illness and possible treatment modalities. The only
requirement of defensive medicine is that the physician take the brief
extra time to record this reasoning process in the medical record. In
fact, the purpose of the medical record is to document the treatment
rendered to the patient so that any future treatment, by the same
physician or by a different health care provider, will have a history on
which to build and benefit the patient. Complete documentation is a
course of action that cannot be criticized; it not only aids defensibility
but, in fact, fulfills the primary purpose of maintaining medical records.

Table 1

General Guidelines[12]

---

1. Adequately, honestly, and reasonably discuss the procedure, its alternatives, its
   risks, and likely outcome with the patient.
2. Give the patient an opportunity to ask questions and answer them.
3. Reasonably document 1 and 2 above, citing at least samples of major risks.
   When the patient has no further questions and accepts the procedure, so indicate.
4. Recognize that exceptions can be used under occasional circumstances, but these
   must be documented at the time. Without such documentation, the retrospective
   utilization of these exceptions may shift the burden of proof to the physician
   and create a significant disadvantage.
5. Pay special attention to informed consent with elective procedures and those
   procedures that have reasonable alternatives.
6. Remember that your record is your best witness. Document!
7. Do not assume the paternalistic role of the past but rather remember the patient's
   right of self-determination and individualism regarding her body integrity.
8. If a complication occurs, honestly inform the patient as soon as possible and
   remind her of your previous discussions regarding risks.
9. Do not alter records.
10. Be aware of local and state case law, legislation, and trends.

References

1. *Ybarra v. Spangard,* 25 Cal 2d 486, 154 P2d 687, 162 ALR 1258, 1944.
2. *Folk v. Kilk,* 53 Cal App 3d 692, 126 Cal Rptr 172, 1976.
3. President's commission for the study of ethical problems in medicine and biomedical and behavioral research. The ethical and legal implications of informed consent in the patient-practitioner relationship (making health care decisions, volume one: report). Washington, DC: US Government Printing Office, 1982.
4. Katz, J. Informed consent—a fairy tale? law's vision. Univ Pitt Law Rev 39(2): 137, 1977.
5. *Mohr v. Williams,* 95 Minn 261, 104 NW 12, 1905. *In* Torts, ed 5, WL Prosser and JW Wade, eds, p 106. Mineola, NY: The Foundation Press, 1971.
6. *Dulieu v. White,* 2 KB 669, 1901.
7. *McCahill v. New York Transportation Company,* 201 NY 221, 194 NE 16, 1911.
8. Roberts, DK Informed consent: a confused and confusing concept. Contemp Ob/gyn 25(5):163, 1985.
9. *Sard v. Hardy,* 379 A2d 1014, 281 MD 432, 1977.
10. *Loudon v. Scott,* 58 Mont 645, 194 P 488.
11. Erickson, SH, Bergman, JJ, Schneeweiss, R, et al. The use of drugs for unlabeled indications. JAMA 243(5):1543, 1980.
12. Roberts, DK. Informed consent and medical-legal problems. *In* Gynecology and obstetrics, JJ Sciarra, ed, chpt 99. Philadelphia: Harper and Row, 1985.

Chapter 10

Nonverbal Communication in the Courtroom

David P. Calvert

The doctor's downcast eyes avoided his patient's gaze. Dr. Smith slowly shook his head and, in a plaintive voice, said, "Bob, I should have known better." The patient's heart sank. He had been through five days of pain and nausea caused by an infection that his doctor said should not have happened. As Dr. Smith listed the reasons for his misdiagnosis, Bob made mental notes for his lawyer.

This scene, which demonstrates the need for accurate communication and gives a preview of the consequences of inaccurate communication, actually happened. The patient received a clear message—the doctor had made a bad mistake and was just waiting to be sued. But the doctor did not communicate his true opinion of what he had done; he communicated only his true feelings. He knew that he had made no errors of judgment, that he had not deviated from the accepted standard of medical practice with his patient, and that there was no basis in fact for a malpractice suit. He had set high standards for himself, and he allowed his anger and disappointment with himself to show.

Ray Birdwhistell, a leading authority on nonverbal communication, states that language accounts for only thirty-five percent of the communication in a two-person conversation.[1] The balance of sixty-five percent is made up of nonverbal signs. Nonverbal communication takes place when all parts of the voice and body are used to communicate—

or even miscommunicate—a message. The trunk, arms, hands, head, face, and eyes all work with the tone and pitch of the voice to give added meaning to the words spoken. Nonverbal messages are most often unconscious. For instance, the person who meets someone for the first time might say to himself, "I don't know what it is about that guy, but I just don't trust him; I don't believe what he said." Such a conclusion probably arises in part from unconscious nonverbal communication—perhaps just a "shifty-eyed look."

Charles Dickens wrote that one of his characters had "affection beaming in one eye, and calculation shining out of the other."[2] Some men are said to have "bedroom eyes"; the "evil eye" is well known; and an angry person is characterized as having "fire in his eyes." Researchers have demonstrated that the pupils of the eye dilate when the individual is viewing something pleasant and contract when viewing something unpleasant. Poker players watch their opponents' eyes to see if they are dilated or not. Other researchers showed photographs of a young woman to test subjects who were asked to indicate which was the most attractive. The photographs were identical but for the size of the pupil, and the overwhelming majority picked the picture with dilated pupils as the most pleasant to look at.

Even more revealing are the facial muscles surrounding the eyes and the mouth. These muscles can cause the eyes to appear squinted, wide open, aghast, frightened, morose, evil, inquisitive, or any number of other expressions. Furrowed foreheads, eyebrow positions, and flaring nostrils tell even more about the meaning behind the words. Added to these cues are the position of the mouth and, if smiling, the type of smile. Nierenberg and Calero report that a British research team has identified nine different types of smiles, ranging from a slight smile (when one is seen as smiling to himself) to a broad smile.[3] Ewan Grant advises people to be wary of the oblong smile—the one that most individuals use when they have to be polite. Most commonly, this smile attempts to convey the idea that the person is paying attention to the conversation but in reality is a million miles away.

Eye contact has also been the subject of intense study. Generally, in a two-person conversation, the conversants look at each other between thirty and sixty percent of the time. When two people are within three feet of each other, a constant gaze by one of those people is threatening and intimidating. Our culture considers the total avoidance of gaze to be a negative indicator. Julius Fast relates the story of a young high school girl who was accused of disrupting activities at school along with two other girls.[1] She was sent to the principal's office and, after a brief conversation during which the girl never looked at the principal and kept her hands folded in her lap, the principal announced his punishment. He told others later that he had deduced her guilt by observing her nonverbal communication. She was guilty because she would not look into the eyes of her accuser. The girl, it so happened, had a reputation for being a cooperative, good girl who would not have done what she was accused of doing. Only later, when the principal explained the confrontation to a friend, did he learn that the girl's cultural background dictated that in order to show respect for her elders she should not look at them when she conversed. He then freely admitted that he had misread her nonverbal signs and rescinded his punishment. The point of the story is that unless the entire background of another is known, there is a chance that nonverbal miscommunication will result.

Because of the possibility of miscommunication, Nierenberg and Calero are careful to point out that gestures do not stand alone—they come in clusters. They may or may not be consistent with the verbal message and should not be taken out of context. No one believes that he has mastered a foreign language if he has only the ability to count to ten and conjugate a few verbs. Even a full understanding of a foreign language does not automatically render one fully capable of engaging in a conversation in that language. The knowledge of what one or two nonverbal signs may mean does not vest one with the ability to read nonverbal communication. As the scenario at the beginning of this chapter indicates, the message received may be totally different from the one sent.

Bedside Manner

The ability of a doctor to accurately send and receive nonverbal communication—although much of it is done unconsciously—not only is the essence of his so-called bedside manner but also can mean the difference between life and death. A multitude of factors influence both the conscious and unconscious messages that a doctor conveys to his patient. Here are a few examples.

A typical picture of a doctor talking to his patient shows the doctor sitting behind his desk, arms folded, leaning back in his chair. The unconscious message is clear. Folded arms are a defensive gesture (e.g., the baseball umpire signals with his arms folded across his chest that his mind is made up and the argument is over); leaning back in the chair indicates an attempt to be as far away from the situation as possible; and the desk is a protective barrier between the doctor and his patient. If the doctor avoids looking at his patient, the patient puts all the signs together and concludes that the news is not good and that the doctor would rather be somewhere else.

In another office, there is no desk between the doctor and the patient; the doctor is just a few feet away. The doctor leans forward in his chair, speaks softly, and looks directly at his patient with his arms uncrossed and hands open. This scene depicts not only the doctor's openness but his desire to establish a communications relationship. There is no sign of trying to shut the patient out. The potential for two-way communication is greatly enhanced when the physical and nonverbal barriers are removed. The way is open for rapport to be established.

Courtroom Manner

Nonverbal communication is equally important within the context of a lawsuit, from the taking of a deposition to the trial in a courtroom. In any given malpractice case, the defendant-physician's objective is to communicate to others the fact that he has not deviated from the standard of care due his patient, if, indeed, he has not. The law is no more an exact science than is medicine. Factors that are unknown and unseen enter into every case, including one called the *YNK factor*— "you never know!" That is, you never know what little things will happen to change or determine the course of a lawsuit. One element of the YNK factor is nonverbal communication.

In almost every malpractice case, the defendant-physician will have his deposition taken. The deposition—testimony given in front of a court reporter with both plaintiff and defense attorneys present—is often taken at the office of the plaintiff's lawyer. Not based on happenstance or convenience, this maneuver is calculated and strategic. Its purpose is to get the doctor on the lawyer's own turf and thus have the upper hand psychologically. Seating the doctor in a low chair is intended to create a feeling of inferiority. The lawyer staring incessantly into the doctor's eyes is calculated to intimidate. During questioning, the lawyer constantly evaluates not only the doctor's answers but his method, manner, and conduct as well. In particular, he looks for such signals as a finger or hand to the lips when speaking, which is considered a sign of deception, as well as gaze avoidance and squirming.

When the case gets to court, the chances of sending nonverbal miscommunication increase along with the chances of misreading others' nonverbal signs. The first opportunity one has to utilize nonverbal skills is during the voir dire—the jury selection process. One attorney recently hired a psychologist to assist him in jury selection. His assignment was simply to observe prospective jurors as they were being questioned and, regardless of their answers to questions, make recommendations based on how they acted. Through the examination of dozens of prospective jurors, the lawyer and the psychologist disagreed on only two of those questioned, giving credence to the theory that lawyers have developed their ability to accurately read nonverbal communication.

The signals indicating who will be favorable jurors and who will not are often clear. Unacceptable jurors clench their fists, cross their arms, and cross their legs. Clearly acceptable jurors lean forward with heads tilted and coats unbuttoned. Those who lean back with hands behind their heads, hands clenched in front of their stomachs, or legs crossed warrant further questioning.

In the courtroom, the defendant-doctor's potential of sending inaccurate signals to the jury is high. With each significant point made or when a witness mentions something the doctor did or said, twelve sets of eyes turn toward the counsel table to see the defendant's reaction. For example, a patient who testifies that the doctor did not tell her about one of the dangers of surgery may prompt the doctor to slowly shake his head from side to side. This reaction can and probably will be read several different ways. One juror may get the message that the doctor is denying his failure to inform; another may think the doctor is wishing the witness had not told the jury of his failure to inform; and yet another may simply see it as a subtle attempt to influence the jury. Nodding the head can likewise communicate different messages. On the one hand, it may indicate agreement with the witness's testimony; on the other, it may be interpreted as an attempt to influence the witness's testimony.

A couple of examples might be instructive. Recently a physician was accused of malpractice by exceeding the scope of the authorization for surgery. He had, in fact, performed necessary surgery, but the patient had not given his permission. The sole issue in the lawsuit was whether or not the patient had given his informed consent. Looking only at the written court record might convince the reader that the award was extremely low considering the facts of the case. However, my interviews with jurors following the verdict convinced me that a number of nonverbal communication factors influenced the amount awarded. The physician's lawyer was pleasant appearing, soft-spoken, and courteous; the plaintiff's lawyer was loud, arrogant, and rude. During the trial and particularly when the doctor's former patient testified, the doctor sat in his chair with both feet on the floor, his coat unbuttoned, as he leaned forward to listen to the testimony against him. The physician's face showed that he was concerned with the welfare of his patient. In fact, when the patient testified about his mental anguish, the expression on the doctor's face seemed to reflect sympathy. When the doctor himself testified, he was totally candid and answered each question directly. The consensus of the jury was that, although the doctor was legally responsible for the damages sustained by his former patient, the defendant was a competent and compassionate physician. This opinion weighed heavily in the doctor's favor.

In two other cases, defendant-physicians nonverbally communicated their attitudes toward their practice of medicine and their patients. In the first case, the doctor appeared in court wearing a rumpled, old-style suit and a tie that almost matched. His careless appearance communicated a careless practice. In the second case, the doctor appeared in a three-piece suit accented by gold jewelry and diamonds. The jury, correctly or incorrectly, saw him as a man interested only in the money to be made from the practice of medicine rather than in his patients.

The defendant-physician should not initiate conversation with his attorney during the testimony of a witness. Any comments should be made on a note pad. There are two reasons: first, the distraction may cause the lawyer to miss some important testimony; second, the jury will see that there is conversation and may draw incorrect inferences about the subject matter.

Demeanor at the counsel table tells the jury a lot over an extended period. The proper demeanor is that of polite attention. Looking around the courtroom, slouching in the chair, and other indications of boredom convey to the jury that the doctor does not consider this case to be important. Such an impression can lead to the conclusion that the doctor has no concern for his patient's problems, whether caused by the doctor's alleged negligence or not. The gestures used consciously or unconsciously at the counsel table can and will communicate the doctor's true feelings to the jury. Almost without exception, people are incapable of maintaining control over their nonverbal communication to the point of completely hiding their inner thoughts, judgments, and feelings.

A witness on the witness stand may also communicate attitudes nonverbally. Jurors, in fact, are generally instructed that they may consider the method, manner, and conduct of a witness in determining the credibility of that witness; in other words, they are encouraged to look for nonverbal signs. The most revealing nonverbal messages are substantially the same as I mentioned earlier. Hand-to-cheek gestures are most often seen as indicating thoughtfulness. Openness and honesty are generally conveyed by open hands, palms up, and an unbuttoned coat. Defensive gestures are arms crossed on the chest, closed hands, fists, or a buttoned vest and coat. Crossed legs, either American style (one ankle on the other knee) or European style (one knee over the other knee), indicate a lack of cooperation. Both feet flat on the floor indicate agreement.

Nierenberg and Calero fully describe these evaluative gestures.[3] During seminars on nonverbal communication, the majority of participants exhibit hand-to-face gestures during the introductory session. Those who are interested in what is being said lean slightly forward; others sit back in a slightly skeptical manner; some cross their arms in defiance; and still others lean forward with elbows on knees and hands open, fully receptive.

These same gestures are significant when they come from the witness stand. A witness turned toward the jury, away from the protection of the witness stand, who sits with his elbows on his knees, leaning forward, will be seen as very receptive to the subject matter of the questions as well as to the examiner himself. The witness who sits close to the stand, using it as a shelf, with arms crossed, legs crossed, and fists clenched will be seen as feeling extremely defensive about the subject matter, the examiner, or both.

There are some other nonverbal signals to be aware of. A tilted head is a receptive, evaluative gesture; when the head is tilted in the same direction as the speaker, it is a sign that things are going well. Some witnesses have what can be called secretive gestures, ones that may appear to be evaluative but in truth indicate suspicion. While putting the hand to the cheek indicates evaluation, the hand to the mouth indicates deception, as if to say "I really don't want to tell this lie." Nose touching and rubbing indicates the answer "No." The person who is really just scratching his nose will rub faster than one who is saying no. Rubbing the eyes and scratching the ears are signs of doubt.

Overall, confident people use far fewer hand-to-face gestures and have more eye contact with others for longer durations. Touching the fingers together in front of the body is called steepling and indicates confidence. The higher the hands are steepled, the more confidence that person has in his position relative to those to whom he is speaking. A judge may steeple his hands in front of his face, while a confident witness may steeple his in his lap.

Sometimes nonverbal communication becomes verbal. I watched one doctor testify on cross-examination for two days. Of the hundreds of questions asked, the doctor answered only about ten percent, although he rarely stopped talking. The message he conveyed to the jury was that he was neither interested in listening to the lawyer's questions nor in answering them. In that particular case, the patient alleged that the doctor did not listen to his complaints and did not explain any procedures to him. The doctor's courtroom demeanor proved the patient's point.

Courtroom communication is strictly one way. The judge, lawyers, and witnesses communicate among each other for the sole benefit of the jury. But the jurors are usually prohibited from any direct verbal communication. In most courts, they may not ask questions of the witnesses or converse with the lawyers. They can and do communicate, however, using nonverbal signs. Although the jury's communication may be unintentional and unconscious, an astute party to a lawsuit can help his lawyer by watching the jurors to see which ones give signs of openness and acceptance as opposed to rejection and defiance. When a witness testifies, he should look at the jurors individually from time to time and try to establish nonverbal rapport with those who are displaying negative nonverbal signs.

Gestures should be read along with all other verbal and nonverbal signs in a conversation to determine consistency. An obvious example of where actions belie the words is the child who is forced to apologize. He may turn his back, walk away, and whisper "I'm sorry" or say it with contempt in his voice. It is abundantly clear not only that he is not sorry, but that he is still angry.

The amateur should use caution when evaluating nonverbal signs, gestures, facial expressions, voice quality, and eye movements. Properly used and interpreted, the art of understanding nonverbal messages can be an invaluable tool. If given too much weight or improperly interpreted, it can lead to miscommunication and perhaps disaster.

References

1. Fast, J. Body language. New York: Simon and Schuster, 1971.
2. Dickens, C. Martin Chuzzlewit.
3. Nierenberg, G and Calero, H. How to read a person like a book. New York: Hawthorn Books, 1971.

Managing the Risk

In a climate where six out of ten obstetrician-gynecologists have been sued (twenty percent three times or more), even the most conscientious medical practitioners will find themselves the targets of litigation. We focus on areas of liability that can be reduced, suggest procedures that can minimize exposure, and give guidelines that can decrease losses. Efforts at managing the risk can eventuate in reducing the number of claims filed, lowering the cost of liability insurance, and allowing physicians' concerns about legal entanglements to return to their proper perspective.

Chapter 11

Practicing Defensible Medicine

Elvoy Raines

The astonishing increase in the frequency and severity of medical malpractice litigation is directly attributable to rising consumerism. Patients are consumers who are concerned about the value of their health care and the services actually rendered. They measure the professional advice rendered and the skills purchased by assessing their quality of life. These patients demonstrate every characteristic of consumers in search of value: investment, expectation, critical evaluation, and accountability. Patients are increasingly using the courtroom to demand that accountability.

The physician predictably responds to the strain, anxiety, and discomfort of being the target of litigation by seeking to avoid the threatening source. He cannot entirely avoid patients, but he can avoid certain patient types. He can eschew certain aspects or obligations of traditional practice, he can limit his exposure by restricting his practice, or he can simply increase fees to a point that appears to make the burden bearable.

Among the changes taking place in the manner physicians practice medicine is one known widely as defensive medicine. The medical community would not criticize defensive medicine if it were good medicine, but the universal conclusion is that defensive medicine equates with ineffective medicine, nonindicated medicine, or, at the least, non-cost-effective medicine. There would be less criticism from consumers and their attorney-advocates if defensive medicine effectively prevented errors of skill or judgment or measurably improved the quality and value of the care provided. But the fact is that defensive medicine is not cost effective, for it exists somewhere beyond the indications essential to justifying action or inaction. Neither does it effectively reduce physicians' exposure to lawsuits. Some argue that defensive medicine, by increasing the risk of complications and poor outcomes arising from the unnecessary procedures themselves, actually increases liability exposure.

To confront the current dilemma of medical professional liability, physicians must adopt a manner of practice that is *defensible,* not defensive. Defensible medicine is a style and substance of practice that is accountable, that can be explained and made rationally comprehensible to nonphysicians. To respond to and correspond with a consumer-oriented health care system, with its gauge of value set to litigate, medical practitioners must clearly make some changes. The issue before physicians is the choice of alternative approaches to practice—either defensive or defensible. It is the purpose of this chapter and the accompanying chapters to explain and illuminate the aspects of defensible practice that are within reasonable bounds of accessibility, within the present capacity and capabilities of practitioners, and sufficiently immediate to deserve consideration for incorporation into everyday practice.

Physicians cannot look to others to cure the problem of medical professional liability, particularly as it besets the specialty of obstetrics and gynecology. Instead, physicians must assume the responsibility and burden of self-education, self-assessment, and self-improvement that can lead to the practice of defensible medicine in its best form. This effort includes understanding basic concepts of law, appreciation of the principles of risk management and incident management, and development of a practice style that evidences a concern for patients' interests that is at least as real as the physician's internalized investment of concern.

Factors in Self-Defeat

Although risk is present in numerous environmental, personal, and institutional conditions, the greatest cause of the physician's liability risk can be found in his own actions. His behavior patterns and practice habits create fertile ground for the actual occurrence of malpractice or, more frequently, the successful allegation of professional performance below acceptable standards.

Even the best and most skilled physicians commit acts in the course of their careers that could serve as the basis for lawsuits. Neither physicians nor their patients can avoid all unexpected outcomes, complications, misunderstandings, and disagreements. However, obstetrician-gynecologists, who perform six or seven of the ten most frequently performed surgical procedures, are exposed to the risk of surgical complications and failures more often than other specialists. Since the complications arising from surgery are the subject of informed consent, physicians must anticipate complications and make contingency plans for the timely recognition of events and the effective management of incidents.

To avoid laying the groundwork for self-defeat, the physician should learn about risk management and attempt to incorporate it into everyday practice. Risk management is not an occasional concern, nor is it an exercise to be performed only with certain patients. Instead, it is a practice style, used in the office and the hospital and so thoroughly a part of practice that the physician grows accustomed to it and eventually does not have to think of practicing in a defensible manner.

Surprise and disappointment are almost always elements of a patient's decision to sue the physician. Through the mechanism of risk management, the physician can avoid surprising and disappointing patients. For instance, a patient who experiences low-grade fever, infection, or an extended hospital stay following surgery is less likely to sue the physician if she is forewarned about the complication or change in expected outcome that becomes reality. The patient will not be disappointed to the same degree when she becomes pregnant several months after a sterilization procedure if she was adequately warned that the procedure does not guarantee sterility. Therefore, the physician who is practicing defensible medicine, who is using an effective process of informed consent, avoids the glaring cases of surprise or disappointment that could occur.

At the foundation of effective risk management—and the avoidance of surprise and disappointment—is the development of communication skills. This concept is so frequently stated that many physicians tend to reject it out of hand as too simplistic, too elusive, or insufficient to prevent lawsuits. But improving communication skills does not mean becoming more chatty, more talkative, and more interesting to patients. Rather, it means that in record keeping, in telephone conversations, in laboratory report interpretations, in consultations, in case reviews, in partnerships, and in surgery, the physician effectively and efficiently conveys the thrust and substance of his message. The notion is not too elusive, because physicians already are trained in observation and articulation of events; they must employ and improve upon these skills in order to actually establish in another person an understanding of that which the physician has observed. Finally, while even the best communication does not absolutely preclude litigation, faulty communication does stimulate successful litigation; inadequate communication does lead to patient injuries; and improved communication does tend to turn aside frivolous or marginal claims.

The busy obstetrical practice is an especially vulnerable setting where ineffective communication encourages litigation. The tendency to over-schedule appointments guarantees delay in seeing patients, elevates their natural level of anxiety, and sets the stage for failures of interpersonal relations that send patients to their friendly attorney for a bit of sympathetic conversation. Naturally, the obstetrician wishes to maximize his productivity and availability to patients, but there is a point of diminishing returns in every practice, and as the obstetrician approaches the point of overload, the risk of error, surprise, or disappointment increases, and so does the risk of lawsuit.

Obstetricians also run considerable risk from failures in communication with other members of the health care team. For instance, there is a difficult pregnancy, and the pediatrician should be forewarned of a potential need for his services at delivery but the message is delayed; problems (such as genital herpes) are discovered during a final office visit prior to confinement, but office records already have been transferred to the hospital; or fetal heart tracings are not retained. These examples all represent important matters that have fallen through the cracks. Although perhaps no actual malpractice occurred, these instances are ones where it is difficult to explain what the physician did and why, problematic to provide an accountability as demanded by the patient, and futile for the physician and his lawyer to try to present in a defensible light.

Defensive medical practice places emphasis upon the potential liability of the physician, often at the expense of good medicine. Defensible medicine gives priority to medical indications and decision making based upon medical training and experience and relegates the legal considerations of medical practice to their proper perspective—important, but secondary to appropriate medical decision making.

Risk Management in Clinical Practice

The individual physician has the ability to control to a large extent his personal risk of liability. The incorporation of risk management techniques into everyday practice is critical to overall reduction of risk. Such risk management begins and ends with the individual physician, but involves the office staff, the basics of the physician-patient relationship, and the special zones of risk inherent in the hospital setting.

A basic, thorough knowledge and understanding of local laws, rules, and regulations affecting practice is essential to risk management. Many physicians do not keep abreast of changing local regulations promulgated by city and state agencies, nor do they become familiar with the working mechanisms of special care programs that have strict guidelines for professional services. The plaintiff's attorney always searches for simple breaches of the rules as a method for attacking the physician's professional performance.

It is difficult and time-consuming to keep abreast of changes in laws and regulations; it is equally burdensome to keep current with developments in the practice of obstetrics and gynecology, especially since it is such a dynamic specialty, changing and developing rapidly. But the expectation of patients as consumers and of courts as arbiters of the standard of care is that every specialist is current in his reading and research and can offer the patient the best care available. The physician can be assured that plaintiffs' attorneys keep up with the medical literature and evolutions in clinical practice.

Specialists share a special risk of liability when they fail to consult or refer. In some instances, this reluctance is based upon the physician's inflated and unrealistic sense of his own abilities—I can do that procedure as well as anyone! But, more often, it is the physician's sincere effort to personally provide final answers and services to the patient that gets in the way of seeking consultations or making referrals. Some physicians want to save the patient the cost of extra professional care; some fear losing the patient to the referred physician; but courts have little sympathy after the fact when a collective approach might have resulted in better care.

A more frequent problem in clinical practice stems from an inadequate cultivation of the physician-patient relationship. The obstetrician-gynecologist normally has a continuing professional care relationship with the woman patient. The physician is that person's principal care physician and treats the whole person. The years of their relationship permit a growth in communication and understanding—the physician's understanding of the patient's personal circumstances and values, and the patient's understanding of the physician's practice style and purpose.

A cultivated relationship prevents many misunderstandings and permits the quick resolution of those that do occur. Such a relationship helps the physician extinguish in the early stages the potential for lit-igation by timely, effective, aggressive response to the patient's disap-pointment or surprise. Some problems arise from simple human frailty or error, such as overscheduling of appointments that lead to delays and anger in the waiting room, or billing errors that insult or confuse patients. These occurrences provide the basis for litigation when the physician is slow or ineffective in his response. In the event of such incidents, timely recognition and aggressive management may be the most critical determinants of whether there will be a lawsuit.

Perhaps the greatest flaw in practice, from the point of view of the risk manager, and the one element that continually appears to com-promise the defense of good medical practice, is poor record keeping. Physicians know how to keep good records. But in a busy practice, the physician tends to take shortcuts, to neglect the recording of routine or clearly understood information, or to have a hasty, sloppy approach that attorneys like to highlight as exemplary of the physician's practice manner. Record keeping is a form of communication: from the phy-sician to himself in the sense of a mental memo; from the attending physician to any other physician who might subsequently treat the patient; from the physician to other members of the health care team to allow them a quick appreciation of the person's condition; and from the physician to patients themselves as a permanent record of the care for which they paid as consumers. In order to maximize the usefulness of this communication tool and thereby to create documentation es-sential to defensible medical practice, records should be clear, legible, factually complete, and recorded in a timely manner.

Much is said and written about changing records, making adjust-ments or corrections in record entries. The frequent mention of this matter springs from the fact that many claims are settled unnecessarily and lawsuits lost because records have been altered, rendering the his-tory of the physician's care indefensible. Alterations or corrections, if not made properly, suggest dishonesty and subterfuge, and compromise the physician's credibility. Therefore, any change should be clearly necessary and fully explained. Corrections must be made chronologi-cally, with reference to the incorrect earlier entry, and then initialed and dated. In that way, anyone reviewing the record (first the plaintiff's attorney and later perhaps a jury) can understand what the physician knew, when he knew it, and how it affected his professional decision making. Corrections may be made but they must be fully explained; however, if the physician has received notice of a claim, no changes whatsoever, even with explanation, should be made after that point.

Special Zones of Risk in the Hospital

The surgical specialties enjoy the dubious honor of being the most frequent targets of litigation. Obstetrics and gynecology, neurosurgery, and orthopedics lead all others in the frequency and severity of lawsuits. The primary reason is simple. When injuries to patients occur in surgery, the impact is likely to be significant and lasting. Those specialists who perform a great deal of surgery increase their risk in sheer numbers of surgical encounters. Over seventy percent of lawsuits involve the hospital as the situs of the alleged injury; therefore, the surgical specialist who uses the hospital to practice his profession should be aware of special zones of liability risk inherent in the hospital setting.[1]

Physicians frequently practice in hospitals unaware of or noncompliant with hospital or departmental rules and regulations. Failure to comply with hospital rules suggests a practice manner below professional standards. Therefore, physicians should know and understand institutional rules and regulations, and comply with their directives. If rules are unreasonable, they should be changed, rather than habitually ignored. It is the responsibility of all physicians to know and comply with the hospital's rules, but the department chairman has a special obligation to review practice records for evidence of noncompliance.

It is prudent for the department chairman and the physicians within each department to meet and agree upon not only rules and regulations but also common terminology, protocols, and lines of authority. The significant interdependence of members of the health care team—from physicians to nurses to technicians to other hospital employees—necessitates a clear understanding of the system to be used in each and every case. Systems and protocols must be periodically reviewed for effectiveness and compliance; records must be randomly examined for completeness and clarity; and evaluations of staff performance must occur in an effort to prevent patient injury and minimize the liability risk of everyone involved as members of the health care team.

Peer review, quality assurance, credentialing, and the process of granting and reviewing privileges are also essential elements in risk management in the hospital. An aggressive program can reduce the risk of injury and improve management of the inevitable but unpredictable poor outcomes.

Technological advances have brought improvements in care and the odds of obtaining desired results, but they have also complicated medical practice and created new zones of risk for physicians. Technological advances have contributed to the elevation of patient expectations, a factor in the creation of disappointment when those expectations are not met. Some physicians argue that the very existence of certain technologies leads to overutilization and unnecessary intervention—consider, for example, the electronic fetal monitor. Furthermore, product liability has had an impact upon physician liability, such as when malfunctions in machinery or systems lead to patient injury; physicians must, therefore, understand and employ mechanisms for the periodic evaluation and testing of technologies in order to anticipate system breakdowns or product flaws.

The importance of the physician's concern and participation in hospital risk management cannot be overemphasized. More than sixty percent of obstetricians have been sued, fully twenty percent sued three or more times, and they are often codefendants with hospitals or other members of the health care team.* As a result of the frequency and severity of lawsuits against the specialty, insurance premiums are increasing at record rates, creating a crisis of affordability for obstetrician-gynecologists. One condition for obtaining hospital privileges may soon be minimum levels of coverage. In some areas and for some physicians, such coverage may be prohibitively expensive or simply unavailable, making it virtually impossible to practice a surgical specialty. The necessity of physicians learning more about risk management should be infinitely clear.

The Solution in Defensible Medicine

Experts in medical professional liability have examined numerous alternatives for solving the professional liability problems that currently beset surgical specialists, particularly obstetricians and gynecologists. Simple approaches, such as changes in law or restrictions on lawyers, have not shown promise in terms of reducing actual patient injuries or limiting the practice of defensive medicine. It *has* been found that physicians who focus their practice style and manner upon the key elements of defensible medical practice—effective communication with patients and other health care providers, thorough record keeping, prudent practice decision making with consultation and appropriate referral, and attention to principles of risk and incident management— actually commit malpractice less frequently, are less threatened by frivolous lawsuits, and more quickly dispatch claims that are pursued.

---

* See Appendix F for a detailed discussion.

Defensible medical practice proves to the potential critic that the physician has performed according to his training and experience, consistent with prevailing standards, and in a manner that best assures the patient and consumer of value for investment. Clearly, defensible medical practice presents the most practical and promising solution to the modern dilemma of medical professional liability.

Reference

1. Raines, E. Survey on professional liability. Washington, DC: American College of Obstetricians and Gynecologists, 1981.

Chapter 12

Common Errors and Prevention

Jeffrey A. Shane

To understand and appreciate some of the problems that may precipitate a malpractice action, physicians should study what has happened in the past, often to competent and conscientious practitioners. Because of some simple or rectifiable error, these physicians have found themselves in claims or litigation that might have easily been avoided had they initially taken a slightly different approach.

Certain things need repetition, and although they may be found elsewhere in this book, they are worth restating. The best defense against malpractice is practicing the best, most current form of medicine. Having done so, the physician must document clearly what was done in the chronological record of care. Before he proceeds to treat the patient, he must make sure that the patient herself and, whenever proper and relevant, other members of her family are active participants in the decision making; and again, this information must be well documented on the chart.

The object is to have a good and defensible chart and not to actually treat the chart. That is, a well-completed chart documents the outstanding medical care rendered and is not just a story of medical care that was, in fact, never delivered. Once he visualizes this concept, the physician is never tempted to try to alter the chart or make other attempts to avoid liability by covering up the facts in a situation. Aside from the ethical (and perhaps legal) restraints upon such conduct, there is also the possibility that it may be discovered, leaving the physician in a more vulnerable, less defensible position.

The common errors that in the past have led to litigation may be divided into the subsections of gynecology and obstetrics. As in other areas, the law has found liability for both acts of omission and commission. An individual may be responsible for failing to do that which he should have done—acts of *omission*—or he may be liable for having done something which he should not have done—acts of *commission.*

Gynecology

Physicians are often the subject of erroneous claims of negligent care, such as when a patient experiences first trimester bleeding, early second trimester bleeding, and spontaneous abortions. Unfortunately, because of the high incidence of first trimester bleeding, and because of the high incidence of first trimester spontaneous abortion, it is reasonable to expect that coincidental events can occur at about the time of such spontaneous abortion which the patient may relate to the fetal loss. If the event happens to have evolved from medical care, then it is highly possible that allegations will be made that the medical care was rendered negligently and resulted in the fetal death. This same syndrome, often seen as a result of an automobile accident or other traumatic event that allegedly caused the abortion, probably accounts for more legal recovery than is reasonably justified. Certainly, the plaintiff who has lost her early pregnancy presents a most sympathetic figure; and for this reason, claims based on loss of pregnancy in the first or early second trimester can never be completely eliminated.

Not every jurisdiction will allow recovery for the wrongful death of an unborn fetus, especially if the fetus was nonviable at the time it was lost. Death actions are, generally speaking, statutory in nature, and the courts look to the definition of *person,* which is usually included in a wrongful death statute, to see whether such definition includes the unborn fetus. Recently a trend has been developing in jurisdictions to allow such causes of action. In addition, even if the estate of the fetus is barred from bringing a wrongful death action, there may very well be cause of action on behalf of one or both of the parents for their emotional distress. In a substantial number of cases, a few minutes spent in the beginning with the patient, giving her a simple explanation about threatened and spontaneous first or early second trimester abortions, will decrease the possibility of a negligence action. The mother who loses a fetus feels a certain amount of guilt, and if it can be explained that the loss was nobody's fault, then a malpractice action may well be averted.

In certain instances, however, the loss of a fetus is a potentially compensable event (PCE). For example, a patient who, during the first trimester of pregnancy, is given drug therapy or is exposed to radiation or some other teratogen, especially on an elective or semielective basis, by the physician who has failed to inquire whether or not the patient is pregnant, may have a valid cause of action for loss of the fetus. Under these circumstances, abortion will often be recommended if the possibility of teratogenesis is significant. In such a case and if such cause of action exists in the jurisdiction, the wrongful death of the unborn fetus is a reasonable claim that may be successfully litigated.

It seems unnecessary to mention to obstetricians and gynecologists that an essential part of any female patient's history is her menstrual history and the possibility of pregnancy, but on occasion even obstetricians forget this simple expedient and expose the unborn fetus to potential teratogenesis. From the point of view of both improving patient care and decreasing litigation, obstetricians must remind all their medical colleagues to question the possibility of pregnancy.

Ectopic pregnancy is an early pregnancy complication that results in a substantial amount of litigation. Ectopic pregnancy still ranks statistically as one of the leading single causes of maternal death in the United States and, therefore, deserves serious respect. Numerous cases arise out of delay in diagnosis or failure to diagnose an ectopic pregnancy. For example, a physician sees a patient with a history either typical or atypical for ectopic pregnancy and sends her home; later she is admitted to another hospital or medical facility when the symptoms become worse or when the ectopic pregnancy ruptures. Under these circumstances, even if the patient does well and has only to undergo a simple salpingectomy, she may allege that earlier intervention might have saved the tube. Allegations are also occasionally made that had the condition been diagnosed earlier, the pregnancy as well as the tube could have been saved. Under these circumstances, one might either look to the second operating surgeon for failing to educate the patient about the nature of the disease process and the treatment modalities for it or to the plaintiff's lawyer's consultant for failing to teach him about the disease process.

The failure to diagnose an ectopic pregnancy becomes much more consequential, however, when the patient undergoes serious physical injury as a result of delay in diagnosis. This may include the need for transfusions with the concomitant risk of hepatitis and possibility of death from exsanguination. When this occurs, the physician is often hard pressed to defend the allegation that the diagnosis of ectopic pregnancy was not given adequate consideration. Without creating a handbook of the myriad ways in which an ectopic pregnancy can be ruled out (e.g., laparoscopy, sonography), it is probably at least sufficient to repeat the adage that once "rule out ectopic" has been included in the diagnostic possibilities, some satisfactory method of indeed ruling it out must be accomplished. The recent advent of such noninvasive techniques as ultrasonography and sensitive pregnancy testing with radioimmunoassay has, on the one hand, made the job somewhat easier and, on the other, made the failure to conduct these tests or otherwise rule out an ectopic pregnancy an area of even greater liability.

Another area with the potential for substantial recovery is the failure to properly evaluate, diagnose, and treat acute salpingitis. Failure to diagnose salpingitis may cause loss of childbearing ability and could be life threatening. Physicians who treat younger patients have extremely high liability in this area. More often, the nongynecologist is the physician who fails to properly evaluate such a condition. One rather common scenario is the patient who has a differential diagnosis of pelvic inflammatory disease or appendicitis—often a difficult differential. However, in evaluating the patient, the gynecologic specialist should be extremely careful to obtain a complete menstrual and reproductive history, even when his initial impression is that the patient has appendicitis. At three in the morning, when the surgeon operates on the patient, finds severe and acute gynecologic infection, and calls his gynecologic consultant back to the operating room, it would certainly be helpful to the gynecologist if he had already obtained the patient's reproductive history and was aware of her future childbearing desires. The operating surgeon, whether gynecologist or nongynecologist, must obtain such a reproductive history from the patient and must explain to her before the surgery begins the possibility that gynecologic disease might be encountered. He must discuss with her the possible alternatives in the event of such a finding and must be aware of just how desperately the patient wants to retain her childbearing ability. To accomplish this matter, the physician simply anticipates the worst finding and includes such a contingency plan in the preoperative discussion. When the patient awakes and finds that a hysterectomy or similar major operative procedure was necessitated, she will be less shocked by the outcome and far less likely to initiate a malpractice action.

Anticipating the worst findings and discussing with the patient the potential alternatives to surgical treatment applies to virtually any operative gynecological problem. Misunderstandings often arise in such similar situations as attempted myomectomy or infertility surgery for chronic inflammation. For example, the physician may determine at the time of surgery that a hysterectomy is necessitated by the nature of the underlying disease. If the physician has prepared the patient by discussing and documenting the alternatives, the patient will be less likely to initiate or to succeed in a malpractice action. The physician must also recognize the patient's right to participate in making this decision that will affect her life and childbearing capacity. Courts and/ or juries often will not accept the notion that the physician is a unilateral decision maker.

In any area of medical practice, the physician who makes promises or warranties about the outcome of a treatment regimen is courting legal action; and he is fooling himself if he believes he can preordain the outcome of even the most minor surgical procedure. A warranty or promise may result in the claim of simple negligence as well as the claim of breach of contract or warranty. Such actions benefit the claimant because there may be no need for expert testimony if, in fact, such a warranty was made. In addition, the statute of limitations for contract actions may extend for a longer period of time than that for a tort action. Thus, the claimant has the means for a successful lawsuit that would not have been available had the physician been reasonable in his expectations and conveyed a reasonable attitude to the patient.

One area of liability which may also initiate a claim for breach of contract or warranty concerns the patient who undergoes elective surgical sterilization. Certainly, the patient must be informed of the possibility that the procedure might fail. If this information is not conveyed or, worse, if sterility is warranted or guaranteed and the patient subsequently becomes pregnant, a wrongful conception action may be brought even in the absence of any negligence in the performance of the procedure itself.* The claim for damages in wrongful conception cases may include the cost of raising the child for a substantial number of years, mitigated to some extent by the benefits derived to the patient from the birth of the child, as well as many other financial losses. If the child is abnormal, especially congenitally deformed or brain damaged, the award can be substantial.

Another area of liability involving either negligence or breach of contract or warranty includes a number of cases arising from dilation and curettage (D and C) procedures, even though few cases have been

---

* These actions may also arise out of other situations such as negligent sterilization and failed abortion.

successful without a showing of negligence. Again, warranties or guarantees must never be made. Even when the anticipated result is virtually
assured and the chance of complications extremely low, preoperative
counseling must include the risk of perforation, bowel injury, and major
surgery from a D and C.

When the procedure being done is to terminate a pregnancy, the
physician can do several things to avoid some of the more common
allegations of negligence. The physician must tell the patient that an
unlikely but certainly possible occurrence is for the operation to fail
and the pregnancy to continue. More important, however, the physician
must be certain that the amount of tissue obtained in an elective termination is reasonably consistent with the estimated duration of the
pregnancy. If the two are inconsistent, he must try to ascertain why by
additional means. Furthermore, he must insist that the pathologist
carefully identify actual fetal tissue or other products of conception and
not simply consider decidua as diagnostic of pregnancy termination.
Of course, there is always the possibility that the pregnancy is extrauterine. When the pregnancy is in utero and continues intact, an action
for wrongful conception or wrongful birth (brought by the parents) or
wrongful life (brought by the child) may result. Pathology specimens
obtained from sterilization procedures must be examined promptly,
and the gynecologist must review the pathology reports and notify the
patient if indicated. For example, the report of one fallopian tube and
one structure consistent with round ligament should prompt vigorous
follow-up of the patient, including immediate notification that the
procedure may have been unsuccessful and that the patient may not
have been sterilized.

The physician who performs a hysterectomy can anticipate a myriad
of complications. Perhaps the single most common operative injury is
damage to the urinary tract system, especially ligation or transection
of a ureter. Whether injury to a ureter during a hysterectomy constitutes
evidence of negligence in the performance of the procedure itself is a
continuing controversy on which there is strongly divided opinion.
Regardless of whether injury to the ureter constitutes care below the
acceptable standard, failure to recognize such an injury and to be
prepared to initiate appropriate emergency therapy is a situation likely
to result in substantial injury to the patient and a high probability of
litigation. The gynecologist who undertakes such operative procedures
in a location where urologic consultation is not available should be
prepared to meet this emergency situation. The patient who develops
a urinary fistula is an extremely unhappy and often truly uncomfortable

patient, one who is likely to allege negligence in her care and treatment. She must receive preoperative counseling about the risk of such an occurrence, even in a simple and uncomplicated hysterectomy.

Obstetrics

No area in medicine carries more risk of potential malpractice liability than the care of the pregnant patient during her prenatal course and delivery. The physician who cares for a young expectant mother also cares for the fetus and newborn infant. Therefore, the physician must be extraordinarily careful in both the obstetric care and in the documentation of this care.

Documentation begins with the first prenatal visit. In addition to obtaining a history and performing a physical examination, the physician must delve into the family history to determine if there are significant risks for the infant (e.g., diabetes). Specifically, the physician must obtain a reasonably comprehensive genetic profile to ascertain whether this child is or might be affected by some congenital anomaly. Although a relatively new cause of action, a number of cases have arisen alleging wrongful life, based on the theory that the child was conceived and born when it should not have been or that the child was damaged by the health care provider's negligence. Several wrongful life cases have been successfully litigated recently. In the first successful case, *Curlender v. Bio-Science Laboratories,* a California appellate court determined that the child could bring an action and be awarded damages for the pain and suffering which she incurred as the result of having been born.[1] In addition, several courts have allowed wrongful birth actions on behalf of the parents for the birth of a child afflicted with a congenital anomaly. In fact, in *Becker v. Schwartz,* the Court of Appeals of New York ascertained that damages were to be the cost of raising a Down's syndrome child for her lifetime.[2] Consequently, such a case carries the risk of significant loss for the defendant-physician.*

Also of great importance is documenting the duration of gestation at the earliest possible moment. This point becomes critical when the physician must deal with the question of prematurity or postmaturity. For the patient whose dates are uncertain, the physician must document early any data indicating accuracy or miscalculation of the gestational age. During the course of the pregnancy, the physician is alert for evidence of developing complications such as toxemia, and obtains early

---

* See also *Turpin v. Sortini.*[3]

baseline studies such as rubella antibody titer in case the patient develops symptoms of a viral syndrome reflecting such an infection.

The physician must obtain from his patient a history of drug ingestion (illicit, prescription, and nonprescription), cigarette smoking, and alcohol intake, and appropriately caution the patient regarding the risk and use of these substances. The patient who takes some medication for other medical problems and who becomes pregnant should be appropriately cautioned regarding any risks of congenital anomalies associated with the particular drug.

Another obstetrical area of potential litigation involves the inadvertent preterm induction of labor or cesarean section resulting in the delivery of a premature infant who suffers respiratory distress syndrome (RDS) and its sequelae. If the physician has not obtained an appropriate history early in pregnancy, it may be extremely difficult to ascertain the maturation of the fetus. Unless the physician can be very certain of the patient's dates, appropriate studies for fetal maturity prior to the initiation of labor or elective repeat cesarean section are strongly indicated in order to avoid a preterm delivery.

The advantages and disadvantages of electronic fetal heart monitoring during the entire course of labor remain controversial, but evaluation of fetal heart tones (FHTs) during the course of labor is essential. FHTs must be recorded at appropriate intervals on the chart. After delivery of a brain-damaged infant, the physician may be able to recall the FHTs; but without physical documentation, the assumption may be made that FHTs were not monitored. The bed sheets sent to the laundry and the scraps of paper discarded with blood pressure and FHTs scribbled on them are of no help; they must be on the chart.

Claims of negligence often surround the attending obstetrician's administration of anesthesia and analgesia. Giving careful attention to total dosages and time intervals, especially with regional anesthesia, the physician delivers the patient with the minimum amount of analgesia and anesthesia required within the bounds of providing adequate patient comfort. The physician who administers a saddle block assumes additional risks. In the event of high spinal or severe maternal hypotension, the physician cannot adequately cope with the problems of both the mother and the infant. He must be assisted by someone who is competent in cardiopulmonary resuscitation, ventilation of the patient, control of hypotension, and any other untoward effect of the anesthetic.

Providing the best medical care for the patient involves availability of the hospital staff and equipment for pediatric resuscitation. Since such teams may not be immediately available, the obstetrician must be competent and trained in newborn resuscitation. Long before the patient is ready to deliver, the physician should inspect the delivery room, making sure it contains adequate pediatric resuscitation equipment, such as functional laryngoscope, batteries, and appropriate size endotracheal tubes.

Conclusion

The optimal way to avoid malpractice litigation is to be optimistic that all will turn out well, while at the same time assuming that the very worst may occur at any time. Foresight in the provision of medical care, preparation for the worst of emergencies, and appropriate risk management prior to catastrophe help to avoid malpractice litigation and provide good medical data for the most defensible case when the truly untoward incident occurs.

References

1. *Curlender v. Bio-Science Laboratories,* 165 Cal Rptr 477 (Cal App), 1980.
2. *Becker v. Schwartz,* 60 App Div 2d 587, 400 NYS2d 119, 1977; *modified,* 46 NYS2d 401, 386 NE2d 807, 386 NE2d 807, 413 NYS2d 895, 1978.
3. *Turpin v. Sortini,* 31 Cal3d 220, 643 P2d 954, 182 Cal Rptr 337 (overruling in part *Curlender v. Bio-Science Laboratories*), 1982.

Chapter 13

Pitfalls Physicians Create
for Themselves

Daniel K. Roberts

In the busy world of seeing numerous patients, many physicians continually fuel the public's criticism of their apparent disregard for rapport with their patients. Physicians' services are in such demand that they forget they are personalized salespeople. Salesmanship plays as much a part in the practice of medicine as it does in the used car business. That does *not* mean selling hysterectomies, tubal ligations, or dilation and curettages (D and Cs). It does mean selling the physician's honesty, his fairness, and probably most importantly his concern for his patients. Why the so-called "quacks" are not sued more often is that they are better salesmen; they sell their concern to their patients. Physicians enter the medical profession because of a basic concern for people. Even in busy office practices, if physicians would spend more time listening to their patients and demonstrating their genuine concern, many, but not all, lawsuits would be prevented. The patient suspicious of her physician's concern will sue more readily.

In the Office

The physician should be concerned about the atmosphere in his office. Is it warm and friendly? Does it emote concern? Do office personnel make the patient feel that she is imposing when she calls for an emergency appointment in an already busy schedule? Do the nurses make inappropriate comments in the hallways? Does the office manager make the patient feel that the sole purpose of the physician's office is to make money to pay for his Cadillac, his swimming pool, his tennis court, or his gambling debts in Las Vegas? Does the patient feel she is being herded through so that the physician can get to the golf course? How does the physician find out? The answer is to ask his patients, either directly or by questionnaire. The physician must ask the questions and then be prepared for some surprises. Subsequent improvement will not only help business but will also reduce the negative atmosphere in which litigation may spawn.

Several years ago, I reviewed the medical records and documents involving four malpractice lawsuits that had been filed against a young, apparently competent, board-certified obstetrician-gynecologist. They all involved postoperative or postpartum care and occurred over a period of seven months. Three of the four suits were unfounded and the fourth was borderline. In spite of the questionable nature of these lawsuits, this apparently high-risk physician was having difficulty acquiring insurance. Investigation determined that one of his nurses not only was making offensive comments in the halls (e.g., "There's nothing wrong with that @#*#@!") but also was treating his telephone calls in a similar manner. She also delayed relaying messages about diagnoses and treatment recommendations for minor postoperative and postpartum complications, angering patients to the point of changing physicians, thus laying fertile grounds for litigation. The physician was unaware of his nurse's behavior at the time. Having a friend or relative make a bogus call to the office once in a while may provide valuable insights into how the office staff supports efforts to maintain patient rapport.

Another aspect of patient-physician rapport concerns full and proper disclosure, known in legal jargon as the doctrine of informed consent. The medical profession has overreacted to this legal notion, which has seldom been the sole issue that determined the success of a lawsuit.* If properly used, it works to the physician's advantage. Full and proper disclosure may deter a lawsuit in the event a disclosed complication occurs. It does *not* protect the physician from a lawsuit if, in fact, the complication is the result of the physician's negligence. The consent

---

* In states that employ a standard requiring disclosure of information that the patient considers material, physicians must be more cautious.

does not have to be lengthy, but the physician must take the time to draft it. As an example,

> I have explained the procedure to the patient as well as its risks and complications (including death, fistula, infections, hemorrhage, etc.). Further, I have offered her the alternatives. The patient indicates that she understands, accepts, and has no further questions.

The inclusion of death and other devastating complications somewhat insulates the physician. If the patient proceeds knowing she might die, have a colostomy, etc., a lesser risk would not likely have deterred her from the procedure.

Although hospital records are frequently incomplete, office records are generally even more often incomplete and unintelligible. I have reviewed office records that ranged from nothing other than the date to "office visit $12," to impossible to read, to very complete and dictated. Physicians are well aware of the difficulties in keeping adequate records as they move through a busy day. In courtroom situations, physicians might wish "If only I had taped her visits," which, of course, is not only impractical but impossible. Certain missing items seem to be important only later when needed as documentation of appropriate medical care.

One of the shortcomings apparent in most medical records is the tendency to list only abnormal findings. Some good examples of omissions that not only occur in a busy office but also assume major proportions in later litigation are:

1. failure to record the size of the uterus and to correlate it with the patient's last menstrual period (LMP) and expected date of confinement (EDC) early in pregnancy;
2. failure to record when fetal heart tones (FHTs) are first heard and when movement is first felt (correlation with dates is once again important);
3. failure to record FHTs on each visit that they are heard;
4. failure to document fundal growth in a systematic fashion and failure to recognize lack of growth and to respond with appropriate follow-up;
5. failure to properly calculate EDC (simple mathematical error) even with an accurate LMP (twenty percent of patients do not

know their LMP and another twenty percent give inaccurate information);

6. failure to record clinical pelvimetry even though it is normal;
7. failure to identify, record, and recognize certain drug allergies;
8. failure to record and recognize certain blood incompatibilities and previous blood transfusions;
9. failure to record and recognize rubella susceptibility with adequate follow-up;
10. failure to record and recognize certain important historical facts such as:
    A. diabetes in the family;
    B. previous large baby;
    C. hypertension;
    D. polycystic kidney disease and other genetic disease;
    E. age of mother (those thirty-five and older require special informed consent regarding antenatal testing);
11. failure to properly respond to and document potential intra-uterine growth retardation (IUGR) problems;
12. failure to recognize the presence or history of genital herpes;
13. failure to recognize previous pelvic inflammatory disease (PID) as a relative contraindication to intrauterine device (IUD) insertion;
14. failure to get a history of the congenital absence of one kidney; and
15. failure to record an LMP or get and record a pregnancy test before D and C or hysterectomy where indicated.

Before leaving this discussion of potential areas of litigation that arise in the office, I want to at least make mention of the following items that deserve the physician's attention:

1. Breast examination is part of the obstetrician-gynecologist's duty. He should not watch lumps grow! He should be extremely conservative and refer early. If a woman feels a lump, the physician should not minimize her concern or pass it off lightly. She may need a xeromammogram or surgical referral to be reassured it is benign.
2. The physician should check Pap smears carefully and not miss an abnormal one. Further, if there are no endocervical cells, he should be aware that it may be an inadequate specimen.

3. The belief that the standard of care concept is being invaded by the bureaucrats and legal profession stems from the case of *Helling v. Carey*.[1] The lower court based its decision on economics, thus affecting what tests are done in the physician's office. The case involved glaucoma and an ophthalmologist who did not perform a tonometry on a thirty-two-year-old patient. The results are best illustrated in the following formula:

IF

B = Burden of providing care
P = Probability, in the absence of care, that injury will occur
L = Likely loss if care not provided

THEN

$B < PL$ = Negligence, even if B is not the standard of care.

4. Another potential area of litigation is the so-called negligent referral concept. The physician may become enjoined in a lawsuit because the quality of his referral was inadequate. Therefore, he should refer his patients to other competent physicians.
5. The physician should not tell his patient that she *must* have a hysterectomy or anything else done. He should give his best and honest advice, the pros and cons, then let her help make the decision. He should never deny the patient a second opinion if she requests it or if he is uncertain.
6. *The physician must not alter records.*

In the Hospital

Hospital patient care presents the physician with problems and concerns similar to those that arise in his office. For example, the physician is again confronted with informed consent, and careful documentation is crucial since surgery is frequently involved. The physician should dictate his operative notes immediately and carefully. If the case has been difficult, he should inform both the family and the patient immediately after surgery to forewarn them of potential complications. The physician should remind them of his presurgery discussion concerning potential problems. If a complication does arise, he should remind them again of their previous discussions. Documenting all discussions in the patient's medical chart is essential.

If a patient's condition warrants, the physician should not only get appropriate diagnostic tests but also call in a consultant. Even though the consultant manages the patient's complication, her personal physician should continue to see her regularly.

Another of the physician's responsibilities is to accurately transcribe the office data about the patient onto her hospital records. For obstetrical patients, accurate and complete hospital records should exist not only for those who are admitted but also for those who have never been officially admitted. For example, the *he-sent-me-home syndrome* is illustrated by the patient who comes to the hospital thinking she is in labor. The physician's medical evaluation based on observation and tests does not support a finding of active labor, and the physician sends the patient home. Later if she delivers a damaged or stillborn infant at home or on the way to the hospital, the patient's recollection is that her physician sent her home in labor. The physician must be certain to explain to the patient that medically she does not appear to be in good labor, that she may go home, but that she should return immediately if her pains get stronger. He must also be certain that the findings of his evaluation, his impressions, and his instructions are recorded.

Once the patient has been admitted, the physician should make sure that the nurses not only are evaluating the progress of labor and the status of the fetus and mother but also are recording these evaluations in the appropriate medical records. For example, recording FHTs is imperative. Several years ago, before a major hospital had a total monitoring system, the department chairman ran a spot check to determine the number of patients who did not have FHTs recorded within fifteen minutes of delivery. Out of forty-seven postpartum patients, twenty-three did not. The FHTs had been taken, but because they were normal and everybody was so busy, they were not recorded. That failure to record data figured prominently in the loss of one and one-half million dollars. In addition to FHTs, it is advisable to record the station and position as well as the FHT. Also, after the birth of the baby, the physician should check the accuracy of the recorded Apgar score with the component scores.

The physician must also recognize the high-risk patient, her needs, and the needs of her baby following delivery. He must know the capabilities of his hospital to handle both the high-risk mother and her child. For example, a common high-risk obstetric patient has a term breech presentation; however, the most appropriate method for term breech delivery is still controversial. Medically there is no question that many can deliver safely via the vaginal route, particularly the frank breech presentation. However, when a brain-damaged infant is born and a cesarean section was not done or given serious consideration and discussion, the resulting lawsuit is frequently settled or lost. I strongly urge a full discussion with the parents. Presented the data, most parents elect cesarean section.

For another high-risk patient, the patient having a repeat or elective cesarean section, accuracy of dates is extremely important. The utilization of other methods such as sonography, lecithin-sphingomyelin (L/S) ratios, and prostaglandin (PG) add support to any case in which prematurity plays a role.

A cost–benefit analysis of electronic fetal monitoring requires monitoring of all high-risk patients during labor and any low-risk patient who becomes high risk. The question of monitoring all patients is somewhat more problematical. The difficulty for the physician is that by the time the case becomes a malpractice lawsuit, the patient and her lawyer, with the advantage of 20/20 hindsight, will indicate that what the physician may have thought was a low-risk patient was, indeed, a high-risk patient. Although some advocate returning to *alle naturale* for a routine delivery, I believe that routine delivery is a postpartum diagnosis. One of the more difficult practical and legal problems is that of appropriate monitor strip record keeping. While it is to the physician's advantage to have as complete and thorough a set of records as possible, storage space is a major problem.

Cultures should be done before antibiotics are given. An extensive family history should be taken. Tests to determine any congenital infectious process should be run. A karyotype should be done if indicated. Early electroencephalogram (EEG) and computerized axial tomography (CAT) scans are frequently helpful. Neurology and cardiology consultations may be of value.

The physician who is named in a lawsuit regarding a brain-damaged infant should have:

1. early evaluation by a *defense* examiner, including a dysmorphologist;
2. chromosome analysis, remembering that a normal chromosome test does not exclude many hereditary-congenital etiologies;
3. tests to include metabolic defects;
4. EEG, CAT scan, skull, bone studies;
5. muscle studies, if indicated;

6. tests to exclude congenital infectious processes;
7. if infant dies, autopsy.

The physician must request timely and appropriate tests to prevent being exploited by the *hypoxia-anoxia-punching-bag syndrome.* An infant may be born displaying symptoms of anoxic injury. Such an infant, however, may be predisposed to anoxic insult before the labor begins because of other etiologies. An alternate hypothesis needs to be developed early and supported by adequate medical documentation.

The *loose-lip syndrome* was exemplified earlier with the nurse who talked too much in the halls of the private office. A second manifestation is frequently seen in labor and delivery and in the neonatal intensive care unit. Some pediatricians, neonatologists, nurses, and medical students have caused litigation to occur by passing judgments and making comments based on partial or inaccurate data. Their intentions are not bad; but because they do not really understand obstetrics, their comments may be devastating. Physicians must be sure to read nurses' notes, just like the plaintiffs' attorneys do!

The physician should not allow technological advances like fetal monitoring to reduce the "laying on of hands" which forged a closeness between the professional and the patient. He must be particularly sensitive to anything that impedes patient rapport, for one of the best defenses against malpractice claims is still a good physician-patient relationship.

Summary

Physicians can help themselves in a number of ways. They can show their concern for their patients and insist their staffs do the same, practice medicine competently, keep patients informed, let them help make decisions, and become knowledgeable about the legal system.

If a lawsuit is filed, the physician must become an active participant with his attorney early. He must be realistic and unafraid to settle if he is wrong. Above all, he must learn to look at lawsuits as the plaintiffs' attorneys do.

As with many other problematic medical therapies, it is wise to refrain from theosophic verbiage, prudent to share the "I don't knows" with our patients, and moral to maintain and fortify every patient's right to self-determination. Yet most importantly, physicians must carefully protect their individual rights, especially from those who would thrive upon the medical profession's inability to provide a perfect therapy when none exists.

Only in these ways can physicians counteract the "ruinous penalties for what the ignorant ignorantly shall decide to be ignorance" (p. xxiii).[2]

References

1. *Helling v. Carey,* 519 P2d 981, 1978.
2. Stryker, LP. Courts and doctors. New York: Macmillan, 1932.

Chapter 14

The Brain-Damaged Child versus the Delivering Physician

Margaret L. Roberts

An obvious lack of oxygen! Add a birth of trauma!
What a perfect setting for the courtroom drama!
This poor child's damage, by the attorney's rendition,
He has found to be . . . the delivering physician!

"Just assume with me," says he now to the jury,
"This defendant-doctor found himself in a hurry.
The fetal heart tones had been long turning sour.
But then, no one had taken them for over an hour."

"And the poor little fetus just couldn't get air.
I guess they all thought he'd had his share.
With CPD, prolonged labor, and an uncaring physician,
You can well image the poor babe's condition."

"Further assume with me, forceps he then did need,
And his hasty extraction caused a cranial bleed.
I'm just a layman, but, my search for the truth
Brings revelation, I've borne the burden of proof!"

"Assume with me . . . ." "I'm just a layman, but . . . ." "Search for the truth . . . ." These familiar phrases, delivered eloquently during deposition or trial by the plaintiff's silver-tongued attorney, are used most often and with the greatest success in cases alleging medical malpractice in the birth of a brain-damaged child. No injury has such a profound effect, both emotionally and financially, on the family, the physician, and society; and, therefore, no area of medical liability can be more easily exploited.

There seems to be a typical pattern of events that surround the birth of a brain-damaged infant and lead to a claim of medical malpractice. An infant is delivered who may be very slightly or gravely depressed. Following resuscitation, if necessary, the infant is taken to the nursery. Unless gross physical anomalies are observed, the admission examination is usually noted to be normal, with the exception of differing degrees of abnormal central nervous system (CNS) response. The infant may have a strange appearance, but subtle dysmorphic features or minor malformations are not likely to be noted. Of course, some brain-damaged infants display the easily diagnosed symptoms and features of a specific, known genetic or congenital syndrome. Quite often, however, there is no absolute, definitive etiologic diagnosis for the infant's CNS disorder. Even so, the admission and dismissal diagnoses are invariably based on the implicit assumption that some avoidable perinatal event is the etiologic culprit, and the medical record contains such phrases as "perinatal hypoxia," "asphyxia neonatorum," "neonatal hypoxic-ischemic encephalopathy," or "birth trauma."

The delivering physician tends to avoid the situation, assuming he may have been able to do something to prevent the outcome. He draws his frustration and emotional distress into his own self-contained shell, attempts to avoid discussing the problem with the parents, and hopes that, by some miracle, the problem will go away.

Neonatal laboratory, pathologic, and radiologic data are often sparse. If specific tests are performed, they usually only verify that a CNS disorder exists, not the time it occurred or the reason why.

The neonatal period is generally spent treating the symptoms that are present. The infant is stabilized and prepared for dismissal. Parental-infant bonding is poor. Both mother and father are in a state of shock, experiencing varying degrees of anger, frustration, and guilt. When they take the infant home, they are frightened and upset. They know they have an abnormal child; seldom do they know the reason why.

Family life is suddenly, totally changed. The parents' dream of bringing home the perfect baby has been shattered. As the child grows, developmental delays are obvious, and care becomes more difficult. As time passes, the frustrations accompanying the constant care of the brain-damaged child increase. No one has yet explained to the family why the child was born this way. The parents' perceptions of the prenatal, labor, and delivery periods become clouded by their growing disappointment, frustration, and hostility. The target begins to narrow down to the obstetrician. He surely could have prevented this tragedy!

Several physicians are generally involved in evaluating or treating the child as it grows. Parents often move or see new physicians in consultation. Most often, the only history noted in the pediatrician's or neurologist's record is one given by the parents—a history that may bear only slight similarity to the one in the actual labor and delivery record. With the passage of time, the labor has become more difficult and prolonged, the contractions much harder, the pelvis considerably smaller, and the delivery more traumatic. For the patient with a history of difficult and prolonged labor, cephalopelvic disproportion (CPD), and/or a difficult forceps delivery, the evaluating pediatrician or neurologist often feels he need go no further. He assumes the child's injury is most probably due to one of those factors. He so states in his record and to the parents.

The parents finally have their answer. They now believe they have confirmation that the delivering physician could have prevented this injury. They proceed to seek legal retribution.

The plaintiff's attorney licks his chops! He has no problem making the diagnosis. He takes the percentage of known perinatal insults, adds the high percentage of unknown and untimed factors, and tops it with the percentage of those problems in morphogenesis the medical profession has failed to diagnose. He assumes the injury was iatrogenic, or knows he has a good chance of making it appear so. He knows that such a grave injury has great jury appeal. Although the records may not reveal anything definitive, he is able to take advantage of an imperfect science, all unknown factors, incomplete and poorly documented records, and prior medical assumptions of etiology. In the name of advocacy, he then forms his version of the truth, his hypothesis of how the injury occurred. His scenario is then presented with the eloquence of his high verbal skills to the defense and jury. The plaintiff's attorney is allowed his inventions because medical science often has no exact answer, and the judge and jury cannot accept such an unsatisfying explanation.

The threat of such lawsuits is not going to disappear. Neither is an instant solution going to be found. Although there is no immediate cure, there is a prescription to palliate the emotional trauma that afflicts the delivering physician. The prescription is learning how to deal effectively with the three major evils that haunt the medical profession—

ignorance, fear, and assumption. The only way to conquer these evils is through individual concern, education, and involvement. Education begins with awareness of all potential causative factors for CNS injuries, including those that are noniatrogenic and those that cannot be recognized prospectively.

Brief Literature Review

In 1862, Little stressed the association of "abnormal parturition, difficult labor, premature birth, and asphyxia neonatorum" (p. 293) with cerebral palsy.[1] Through the years, little thought or attention was given to potential antepartum etiologic factors. Most of the writing of the 1950s reflected the opinion that perinatal insults were the predominant etiologic factors in cerebral palsy. This opinion still permeates present-day clinical thinking, to the distinct advantage of the plaintiff community. It survives side-by-side with the knowledge that although the techniques and practice of obstetrics have vastly improved in the past thirty years, the incidence of cerebral palsy has not shown an appreciable decrease.

Warkany makes the point that infants with prenatal injuries can be asphyxic at birth and be born of difficult labors.[2] He further states that, as obstetrical factors lose some of their relative importance, prenatal factors come to the foreground and assume a more prominent role among the causes of cerebral palsy. Towbin also supports the concept that there are instances of in utero asphyxia which are not preventable: "There is pathologic evidence that a major portion of CNS lesions present at birth are due to latent processes having origin prenatally and may be well advanced prior to labor" (p. 529).[3]

Volpe describes a variety of CNS lesions which present as neonatal hypoxic-ischemic encephalopathy.[4] The neuropathological features vary considerably with such things as the gestational age of the infant, the nature and timing of the insult, and the type of interventions. Studies were reported which showed the vast majority of infants who presented with this clinical picture were those who experienced intrauterine asphyxia. Of those, the higher percentage were felt to have experienced the principal insult during the antepartum period.

In the Collaborative Perinatal Project, one-minute and five-minute Apgar scores for 14,115 children were studied and used to predict neurological deficits in children at one year of age.[5] The one-minute score identified the effect on the fetus of anesthesia and analgesia used

Table 1

One-Minute and Five-Minute Apgar Scores as Predictors of Neurological Deficits in Children at One Year of Age

Neurological Assessment	One-Minute Apgar Scores			Five-Minute Apgar Scores			Total
	0–3	4–6	7–10	0–3	4–6	7–10	
Abnormal	3.6%	2.8%	1.6%	7.4%	5.3%	1.7%	1.9%
Normal	96.4%	97.2%	98.4%	92.6%	94.7%	98.3%	98.1%

during labor and delivery. In addition, it identified the neonate requiring resuscitation and was a useful predictor of neonatal mortality. Because the child's condition may change rapidly in the first few minutes of life, five-minute scores were routinely obtained. The data in Table 1 strongly indicate that, irrespective of birth weight, the five-minute score is a useful predictor of neurologic impairment. Researchers noted that it was impossible to know whether a low one-minute and five-minute score were expressions of already abnormal children or whether pathophysiological mechanisms underlying the low scores were responsible for the impairment. In consideration of the overwhelming percentage of infants with low scores who were later found neurologically intact, there is certainly the strong possibility that those infants who were later diagnosed as having lasting CNS abnormalities were those whose perinatal insults were superimposed on primary antepartum insults.

Myers, the most prolific writer on the experimental production of brain damage subsequent to maternal hypoxemia and fetal hypoxia-asphyxia, evaluates the overall spectrum of oxygen deprivation and the associated consequences to the fetus.[6]

> When the marked severity of the asphyxia that is required to produce brain injury is considered along with the necessity of its enduring for the required length of time, it is apparent why survival with brain damage due to asphyxia is relatively uncommon and why sudden death or an apparently intact survival are much the more likely outcomes of intrauterine asphyxia [p. 55].

Utilizing records of 17,265 cases selected from the population of the Collaborative Perinatal Project, Niswander, Friedman, and Berendes analyzed the neurologic development at one year of over 300 children exposed to obstetric emergencies thought to be potentially hypoxigenic, i.e., abruptio placentae, placenta previa, and prolapse of the umbilical cord.[7] They concluded that perinatal hypoxia as evidenced by these pathologic conditions may not be a potent cause of brain damage as tested by motor function, provided the child's birth weight was in the mature range.

An additional study was subsequently performed, utilizing a new protocol designed to avoid potential bias of the previous investigation and to extend the neurologic follow-up to four years.[8] They concluded that, excluding those children of low birth weight, intrauterine hypoxia-asphyxia apparently is not a major cause of neurologic dysfunction in the surviving child.

Niswander discusses the fact that perinatal asphyxia as a cause of brain damage is currently in vogue with trial lawyers, and that it is almost a reflex reaction to blame the delivering physician for any infant born with CNS dysfunction.[9] He states, "The scientific basis for relating perinatal asphyxia to subsequent brain damage in an individual patient is tenuous at best" (p. 358).

In 1980, Haesslein and Niswander reported the results of a study including 3,972 term deliveries.[10] The study was performed to determine:

1. the frequency with which electronic fetal monitoring (EFM) over-diagnosed or underdiagnosed fetal distress;
2. the frequency with which the distressed fetus had a major congenital anomaly;
3. whether the time lapse between the diagnosis of acute fetal distress and delivery was a critical factor which controlled the degree of risk of brain damage; and
4. if there were identifiable prenatal factors, which in combination with an abnormal EFM tracing, predict an increased risk of neurologic damage.

In the study, they found:

1. The EFM tracing classically thought to indicate fetal distress was wrong about seventy-five percent of the time as judged by a five-minute Apgar score of less than seven. In ten out of 3,972 term infants, an entirely normal EFM tracing was followed by an unexpectedly low five-minute Apgar score.
2. Congenital anomalies were present in less than ten percent of the term infants who were diagnosed as distressed in utero.
3. The time allowed to elapse between the presumed diagnosis of fetal distress and delivery seemed to be less crucial to the neurologic outcome of the fetus than was the presence of evidence of *chronic* fetal distress.

4. They concluded that evidence of perinatal asphyxia was not followed by neurologic abnormality of the infant unless there was
preexisting chronic fetal distress.

In 1980, a placental lesion associated with fetal mortality-morbidity
was discovered and described by Sander, a Michigan pathologist.[11] The
lesion, hemorrhagic endovasculitis (HEV), is of unknown etiology and
marked by the insidious fragmentation of erythrocytes and destruction
of vessel walls in discrete sections. Other laboratories have verified the
fact the lesion exists. Sander, who examines placentas associated with
problem births from all over Michigan, determined early in his research
that fifty percent of fetuses involved were stillborn and that a number
appeared to have experienced fetal distress. Of the 3,500 problem
placentas examined, nineteen percent or 700 have shown the lesion.
With half of the cases stillbirths, HEV may have blighted hundreds of
survivors of problem births. In many HEV cases, Sander has detected
a villitis characteristic of the TORCHS group of viruses.* Several of
the mothers have now given birth to second HEV babies. Sander has
begun an overall epidemiologic study, also taking a closer look at HEV
mothers, focusing on their endocrinologic, immunologic, and vascular
status.

In 1982, Holm reported a retrospective study of 142 children with
cerebral palsy.[12] He found prenatal causes in fifty percent of the cases,
perinatal causes in thirty-three percent, postnatal causes in ten percent,
and mixed causes in seven percent. Holm comments, "The finding in
this study that 50% of cerebral palsy is of prenatal origin is, if anything,
an underestimate" (p. 1473).

At the 1984 western clinical research meetings held by ACOG, Lindenberg presented data showing prenatal brain damage occurs more
often than suspected in both term and preterm infants.[13] In the study,
autopsies were performed on forty infants during a one-year period;
the duration of the injury was estimated by neuropathologic assessment.
Of those autopsied, thirty-one infants (twenty-five preterm and six term)
died during the first week of life. Six of the twenty-five preterm infants
showed evidence of prenatal brain damage, and four of the preterm
infants were felt to have a markedly low level of brain maturity for
their gestational age. Five of the six term infants showed evidence of
prenatal brain damage. Lindenberg reported that two of the five term
infants and seven of the ten preterm infants with prenatal brain pathology had low one-minute and five-minute Apgar scores. Of the term

---

* Toxoplasmosis, Other, Rubella, Cytomegalovirus, Herpes, Syphilis.

infants, the two with the earliest injuries had the lowest scores. Lindenberg stated the results suggest that infants with prenatal brain damage do not tolerate labor well; however, he noted that fetal distress was severe enough to warrant cesarean section in only three cases.

In October 1984, Niswander et al. reported the results of a study, the purpose of which was to determine the relationship between four possibly preventable adverse outcomes of pregnancy and suboptimal antepartum and intrapartum obstetric care defined by clinical consensus.[14] Cases and controls were derived prospectively by the Oxford Cerebral Palsy Study from 16,400 babies delivered at the John Radcliffe Hospital in Oxford, England, between January 1, 1978, and December 31, 1980. From those deliveries, the following categories and case series were extrapolated and studied:

1. fetal deaths ascribed to asphyxia or trauma, case series of fifty-eight (3.5 per 1,000 births);
2. terminal apnea, case series of ninety-two (5.6 per 1,000 live births);
3. seizures within forty-eight hours of birth at term, case series of thirty-six (2.2 per 1,000 live births); and
4. cerebral palsy, case series of thirty-four (2.1 per 1,000 live births), provisional diagnosis made at eighteen months of age.

Without knowledge of the condition of the infant at birth, the obstetricians closely examined the clinical records to assess the quality of obstetric care. Pediatricians, experienced in neurological examination of the newborn, scrutinized the records of all babies reported to be neurologically abnormal at any stage of the neonatal period. In addition the examinations of the children with cerebral palsy were made by a pediatrician who had no knowledge of the perinatal history. From the available data, the study concluded:

1. Fetuses whose deaths were ascribed to asphyxia or trauma and babies born at term who had seizures within forty-eight hours of delivery were significantly more likely than controls to have received suboptimal care during pregnancy.
2. Babies with seizures, as well as those with terminal apnea, were also substantially more likely than controls to have been born after a failure to react appropriately to signs of severe fetal distress during labor.
3. Most of the babies who received suboptimal care, however, did not have any of these adverse outcomes.

4. Most babies with these adverse outcomes had apparently received satisfactory obstetric care.
5. No relation was detected between cerebral palsy and suboptimal obstetric care.

Considering the overwhelming numbers of dollars which have been awarded to plaintiffs in cases involving brain-damaged children, the opinions and studies discussed here are certainly suggestive that the obstetric community has been bearing the burden of assumption, rather than proof. Both the differential diagnosis and treatment of the malpractice malady have been poor.

Discussion

The high percentage of injuries of unknown etiology evidences a fact that the plaintiff community has used to their advantage in the past—that medical science is imperfect and in a constant state of change. The delivering physician must be aware of the increasing data showing that factors present in the prenatal period may be responsible for abnormalities or for predisposing the infant to problems which may become manifest during the labor, delivery, and neonatal periods. The explosive growth of genetics, teratology, and dysmorphology are resulting in the description of new malformation syndromes. The presence of clusters of dysmorphic signs is now recognized as a marker of disturbed prenatal development. A careful look at the cerebral palsy population reveals children with syndromes only recently described, as well as children with enough dysmorphic features to represent as yet undiagnosable syndromes.

The delivering physician must further familiarize himself with his rights and responsibilities within the legal context. He can then stop fearing the law and start making it operate for his benefit.

If a brain-damaged infant is born, the delivering physician must not ignore the problem. He must keep the line of communication open with the parents. To do otherwise gives the appearance that he is assuming guilt. Although he is uncomfortable with the unfortunate outcome, the parents are profoundly affected and are experiencing the day-to-day distress that may subsequently culminate in a legal action.

The delivering physician must enlist the aid of the attending pediatrician, pediatric neurologist, geneticist, and others caring for the infant during the neonatal period. He must give them an accurate history of prenatal, labor, and delivery events. He should request that pertinent clinical examinations and testing be performed to rule out any potential genetic or congenital factors that might have resulted in the injury. Should a legal action subsequently be filed, an accurate etiology may be difficult to obtain retrospectively.

If a lawsuit is filed in spite of preventive measures, the physician should become actively involved in his own defense. He needs first to establish a good relationship with his defense attorney, making every effort to be open and honest in all aspects of the case in question. At the same time, he should expect to receive an informed consent of the same quality he is expected to give a patient. In this manner, he is a knowledgeable participant during each stage of his own legal "treatment."

The physician must not assume, nor should his attorney assume, that causation for the injury is as alleged by the plaintiff. If a thorough medical examination and evaluation of the child has not been performed, he should request that such be obtained.

Evaluation for the Defense

Many cases involving a brain-damaged child never reach the courtroom. Unfortunately, they are settled before thorough claims analyses and evaluations are made, before all alternate hypotheses have been explored, and before thorough medical evaluations have ruled out any possible genetic or congenital factors. Therefore, before any legal action is settled or taken to trial, the defense must require a thorough medical examination and evaluation.

To perform the evaluation, the defense must assemble a team of experts. A *claims analyst* evaluates and summarizes all available medical records as well as all data obtained during the discovery period. An expert *obstetrician* not only reviews the claims analyst's evaluation and summary, but also examines and evaluates all records pertinent to the care and treatment provided prenatally and during the labor and delivery period, considering all potential high-risk familial, maternal, and fetal factors. A *neonatologist-pediatrician* examines the child after reviewing the claims analyst's evaluation and after examining and evaluating the pertinent neonatal and pediatric records. A *pediatric neurologist* also examines the child and supervises additional tests, after becoming familiar with the claims analyst's evaluation and the pertinent neonatal and pediatric records. A *pediatric geneticist,* following a review of the other experts' analyses and the pertinent records, interviews the parents to elicit a thorough history of the family pedigree, examines the child for all possible major or minor malformations suggestive of problems in fetal morphogenesis, and supervises tests to rule out genetic or congenital factors.

A complete evaluation of the child will likely entail a two- to three-day hospitalization. Tests recommended include:

1. karyotype, to rule out any chromosomal abnormalities;
2. metabolic studies, to rule out inherited metabolic disease;
3. CAT scan, to determine the presence or absence of CNS pathology;
4. EEG, if indicated;
5. muscle studies, if indicated;
6. skeletal survey;
7. child development evaluation, to include hearing, sight, speech, etc.; and
8. other tests as indicated after examination.

When the medical testing and evaluation is complete, all parties involved in the evaluation meet to discuss the most probable etiology for the child's injury. At this conference, they should answer the following questions:

1. Does the injury reflect traumatic insult?
2. Does the injury reflect an hypoxic-ischemic insult? Diffuse or focal? In what specific areas?
3. Do the records and evaluations reflect possible fetal predisposition to the injury?
4. Does the evaluation of the injury reflect possible genetic or congenital involvement?
5. Does the evaluation of the record and type of injury reflect iatrogenic involvement? If so, do the records and evaluation indicate whether or not the injury could have been recognized and avoided prospectively?

During the conference, these experts should discuss all alternate etiologic possibilities for the child's injury. Even if this group of experts cannot determine the probable or actual etiology or cannot ascertain whether medical deviation occurred, this final opinion is valuable to the defense.

Conclusion

Recall the three favorite phrases of the plaintiff's attorney. Understand why they have been used so successfully by the plaintiff in the past and how they can be surmounted successfully by the defense in the future.

"Assume with me . . . ."

With continued education and understanding of available research data, the medical community must learn to assume nothing. Ignorance and fear breed assumption which, in turn, may continue to breed injustice. Observations and opinions that are based on assumption and that bear false conclusions aid the metastasis of the malpractice malady, slow the progress of medical science, and provide precedents that breed further injustice.

"I'm just a layman, but . . . ."

The plaintiff's attorney is *not* an ordinary layman. Specific texts and courses train attorneys in the specialty of obstetrics and advise them about how to proceed and how to effect victory. The delivering physician must likewise acquire knowledge of the legal system, so he does not find himself at a disadvantage when in the unfamiliar legal arena.

"Search for truth . . . ."

With the knowledge that truth is relative and that some injuries still defy definitive diagnoses, the medical community must begin to take advantage of its own resources, which remain almost untapped. At the same time, plaintiffs' attorneys must not be allowed to project superior medical knowledge in areas the science itself has yet to comprehend. Without physicians' direct concern, education, and active involvement, the final diagnoses of brain-damaged children will continue to be made in the courtroom by plaintiffs' attorneys.

Although it seems that the delivery of a brain-damaged child is synonymous with legal action, obstetricians must never lose sight of their first and foremost goal—true concern for those patients whose lives have been entrusted to them, both mother and fetus. Ignorance, fear, and the assumption of guilt have too long overshadowed logic and, as a result, have cast both patient and physician in a losing role.

The physician who fails to gain knowledge of, to consider, and to explore the abundant number of noniatrogenic injuries impedes the progress of the science. Each delivering physician has a duty to lay the foundation for the science and, in the process, to reap the reward of an honest and scientific, rather than a legal, search for the truth.

Editorial Note

As this book was nearing the final stages of publication, a National Institutes of Health panel released the findings of recent studies which may prove to be a major breakthrough in the defense of cases involving brain-damaged children. In a 450-page report, the panel of ten leading child development experts concluded: (1) that brain damage among newborns is usually *not* caused by physician negligence; and (2) that in the vast majority of cases, the specific cause is not known and, therefore, blame cannot be assigned. The editors urge the reader to review the specifics of the report when it becomes available.[15]

References

1. Little, W. On the influence of abnormal parturition, difficult labours, premature birth, and asphyxia neonatorum, on the mental and physical condition of children, especially in relation to deformities. Trans Obstet Soc London 3:293, 1862.
2. Warkany, J. Congenital malformations. Chicago: Year Book Medical Book Publishers, 1971.
3. Towbin, A. Central nervous system damage in the human fetus and newborn infant. Am J Dis Child 119:529, 1970.
4. Volpe, JJ. Neurology of the newborn. Philadelphia: WB Saunders, 1981.
5. Drage, JS, Kennedy, C, Berendes, H, et al. The Apgar score as an index of infant morbidity: report from the collaborative study of cerebral palsy. Develop Med Child Neurol 8:141, 1966.
6. Myers, RE. Experimental models of perinatal brain damage—relevance to human pathology. *In* Intrauterine asphyxia and the developing fetal brain, L Gluck, ed, Chicago: Year Book Medical Book Publishers, 1977.
7. Niswander, KR, Friedman, EA, and Berendes, H. Do placenta previa, abruptio placenta and prolapsed cord cause neurologic damage to the infant who survives? *In* Studies in infancy (clinics in developmental medicine, no. 27), R MacKeith and M Bee, eds. Suffolk, England: Lavenham Press Ltd, 1968.
8. Niswander, KR, Gordon, M, and Drage, JS. The effect of intrauterine hypoxia on the child surviving to 4 years. Presented by invitation at the eighty-fifth annual meeting of the American Association of Obstetricians and Gynecologists, Hot Springs, Virginia, September 4–7, 1974.
9. Niswander, KR. The obstetrician, fetal asphyxia and cerebral palsy. Am J Obstet Gynecol 133:358, 1979.

10. Haesslein, HC and Niswander, KR. Fetal distress in term pregnancies. Am J Obstet Gynecol 137:245, 1980.
11. Medical Tribune 25(8):1, March 21, 1984.
12. Holm, VA. The causes of cerebral palsy: a contemporary perspective. JAMA 247:1473, 1982.
13. Lindenberg, J, Goetzman, BW, DiNello, C, et al. Calls for assessing prenatal brain damage. Ob Gyn News, April 1–14, 1984, p 1.
14. Niswander, KR, Elbourne, D, Redman, C, et al. Adverse outcome of pregnancy and the quality of obstetric care. Lancet 2(8407):827, 1984.
15. Freeman, JM, ed. Prenatal and perinatal factors associated with brain disorders. Washington, DC: National Institutes of Health, 1985.

Chapter 15

Claims Analysis

Margaret L. Roberts

Once a claim has been made, a thorough, well-prepared analysis of that claim is one of the finest tools available to the insurance company, the defense counsel, and the potential defendant-doctor. A detailed, complete evaluation of the medical records may be the instrument by which the claim is eventually dropped, a lawsuit subsequently dismissed or settled, or an action finalized by a favorable disposition for the defendant-doctor. Although there are numerous differences, the general method of the analysis is applicable to both the gynecologic patient and the obstetric patient. A thorough claims analysis includes: (1) chronological documentation of the medical data, (2) observations regarding the medical data, (3) alternate hypotheses, (4) claim summary, and (5) scientific data to support conclusions. When a case goes to trial, the claims analyst generates documents that organize and detail a medical chronology to follow, the allegations and issues to address, and the medical-legal points to establish.

Chronological Documentation of Medical Data

The medical data that are immediately available after a claim is filed are often sparse and incomplete. An evaluation based on incomplete data results in an incomplete evaluation. Medical records ideally include documentation from:

1. prior office visits and hospitalizations that may be pertinent to the present claim;
2. office visits and hospitalizations that involve the patient's complaint, diagnosis, and treatment from which the alleged injury resulted; and
3. office visits and hospitalizations following the alleged injury that may be pertinent to the present claim.

These records document the patient's medical history as well as her family's history. The history a patient gives to one physician is not always complete. Histories given to other physicians or given at the time of hospitalizations often provide additional data.

Once all the available medical records are in hand, the task is to extract specific data and organize it chronologically. With the data in the appropriate time sequence, patterns may emerge that not only can provide valuable information regarding the alleged injury but also can help determine whether the injury could have been prevented.

Observations

Before making observations regarding the documented medical data, the analyst examines the subjective and objective data that the physician possessed. The analyst then assesses both the data and the plan for treatment. Considering the subjective and objective data available to the physician, the analyst answers the following sets of questions:

- Did the diagnostic method used comply with an appropriate standard of practice? Was the chosen treatment within the medically approved standard? If not, did the diagnosis and/or choice of treatment involve a judgment call or did it deviate from the medical standard?

- Did the patient's past medical history suggest circumstances that might have precluded a good result? Were they known prior to the procedure? Should they have been known prior to the procedure?

> Following a vaginal hysterectomy, during which time her legs were in stirrups, a patient experienced a temporary peripheral neuropathy in the form of a unilateral foot drop. She alleged that the precaution of providing sufficient pad-

ding had not been taken during the procedure to prevent such an occurrence. A neurologist was subsequently consulted. During his workup, he discovered the patient had diabetes, a condition to which he attributed the postoperative problem. The medical record revealed that the patient had not given a history of diabetes and that routine, preoperative laboratory work had not discovered the disease. Therefore, the treating physician could not have known prospectively that the patient was at high risk for this complication.

- Was the patient made fully aware of her condition? Did she understand the choice of treatment, the alternatives, and the risks and complications that might result? Did she concur in the decision to proceed with the treatment?

- Was the patient negligent by failing to follow recommendations, take medications appropriately, and/or return for further diagnosis and treatment?

> In the case involving foot drop, the patient had failed to keep appointments for physical therapy. Had the lawsuit been pursued, she would have had difficulty convincing a jury that her injury was very serious.

- If the treatment was surgical, was the procedure performed in accord with the medically approved standard of practice? Did the findings at the time of surgery and/or the surgical pathology report verify the preoperative diagnosis?

- If the alleged injury occurred during a surgical procedure, were circumstances present that could have precluded an optimum result, e.g., massive adhesions, carcinoma, or other unexpected findings?

> During a routine postpartum tubal ligation, the physician perforated the patient's bowel. She subsequently developed peritonitis and required additional surgery and an extended hospitalization. During the second surgical procedure, the physician discovered the patient had a congenitally malrotated bowel, a condition that contributed to the perforation.

- Was there a deviation from the medical standard of practice by hospital or laboratory personnel, by blood bank or surgical pathology technicians, or by consultants?

  Prior to a repeat cesarean section, the laboratory erroneously reported a mature lecithin/sphingomyelin (L/S) ratio. Following delivery, the neonate experienced an extended hospitalization while successfully recovering from respiratory distress syndrome (RDS), a condition that could have easily been avoided.

- When complications occurred, were they appropriately recognized and treated? Were they documented? Was the patient and/or family informed?

  After a normal course of labor, a young primigravida uneventfully delivered her infant. Following delivery, the patient was taken to her room. Although the uterus remained firm, the nurse's notes revealed that during the next few hours the patient experienced a significant amount of bleeding. The notations also indicated that the patient's blood pressure was slowly decreasing and her pulse was slowly increasing. She became diaphoretic and increasingly restless. By the time the decision was made that blood and fluid replacement were needed, the patient's veins had collapsed. She died a short time later. This death could easily have been prevented by a routine postpartum examination of the patient's cervix and vagina. She had slowly, literally bled to death from lacerations that could have been repaired following the delivery.

- Are the medical records complete? Do they include all data necessary for a complete and thorough evaluation? These are:
  1. history and physical examination report;
  2. physician's orders;
  3. physician's progress notes;
  4. consultants' reports;
  5. laboratory, pathology, and radiology reports;
  6. medication charts
  7. vital signs charts;
  8. nurses' notes;

9. summary sheet; and
10. discharge summary.

- Have any of the records been altered?

  A case was filed regarding an infection that occurred following an abdominal hysterectomy. The complication was recognized and appropriately treated. The patient's hospitalization was only briefly extended. The records indicated no evidence of medical deviation on the part of the treating physician. In addition, postoperative infection is a known complication of such a procedure. The records did reflect, however, that documentation of the patient's informed consent had been written into the record at a later date. The doubt that was cast on the physician's integrity effected a small, but unnecessary settlement.

- What was the extent of the injury? Was it temporary or permanent? Was it one requiring a short period of hospitalization, one requiring an extended period of hospitalization, or one requiring additional hospitalizations? Did the injury involve the central nervous system and/or result in death?

Evaluation and observations regarding claims involving obstetric patients require special consideration. The physician is providing care and treatment for both mother and fetus, and the outcome is dependent on a multitude of factors that start with the genetic heritage and evolve through conception, implantation, gestation, labor, and delivery. Any of these factors may potentially be affected by both intrauterine and extrauterine events. In attempting to ascertain whether an obstetric injury or loss could have been prospectively recognized and prevented in the particular case under scrutiny, the claims analyst concentrates on: (1) the family history, (2) the prenatal record, and (3) the labor and delivery record.

Family History

The entire family history is important. Although it is the mother who is providing the intrauterine environment for the fetus during the most important period of development, the final product is the sum total of all past generations. Family histories have a tendency to change after a lawsuit has been filed. Aunt Nellie, who was once noted as being mentally deficient at birth, is reported to be in perfect health during deposition; and Cousin Christopher, who was once noted as experiencing seizures of unknown etiology from the time of birth, is later reported to have been injured in a fall from his little red wagon at the age of three. Therefore, family histories given prior to filing often reveal loose limbs of the family tree that can be documented before the pruning ceremony takes place during deposition or trial.

The patient's complete medical history from her birth to the time she requests prenatal care is important. It should include details about past and present menstruation, contraception, pregnancies, chronic illnesses or medical conditions, nutritional state, and exposure to drugs, alcohol, and cigarettes. Such a history identifies the high-risk factors that may have been present at the onset of pregnancy and those that may have developed during the gestational period.

Prenatal Record

The prenatal record provides data about fetal environment, growth, and development before labor and delivery. The analyst can determine whether or not evidence of potential problem areas existed by examining laboratory data, clinical pelvimetry, and clinical notations regarding maternal weight gain, measurements of urine glucose and albumin, blood pressure, presence of edema, abnormal bleeding, infection, fundal growth, etc. The length of gestation is often questioned in obstetric claims, making it important to note the accuracy and quality of the last menstrual period (LMP), the size of the fundus at initial examination and the growth pattern thereafter, the time of quickening, the initial presence of fetal heart tones (FHTs), and any sonographic examinations.

Labor and Delivery Record

Most obstetric claims arise from events that happen during the labor and delivery process. Therefore, the record of the difficulties that occur during labor and delivery or the documentation of the maternal or fetal problems which are present before the onset of labor that become manifest during labor are of utmost importance to an analysis of the claim. Following are some of the critical sets of questions that must be answered in determining the merits of the case.

- Since the initial admission assessment of both mother and fetus can identify potential problems, were the high-risk factors that were present prenatally noted on the chart? Was there any initial evidence of potential problems from the admission laboratory data, maternal vital signs, status of membranes, onset of regular contractions, quality of contractions, fetal heart tones, fetal stations, and presentation?
- Did the length of the latent and active phases of the first stage of labor indicate possible protraction or arrest disorders? If an abnormal pattern occurred, what assessment was made in regard to the etiology of the dysfunction? What treatment was initiated? Was such treatment appropriate? Was the second stage of labor normal?
- If an oxytocic agent was utilized, what were the indications or contraindications for the drug, the amounts given, and the quality and frequency of the contractions thereafter? What assessments of fetal well-being were made during that period of time?
- If analgesic or anesthetic agents were used, were they given at appropriate times and in appropriate amounts? Was there any abnormal maternal or fetal response?
- Of paramount importance is the assessment of fetal well-being during the entire course of the labor and delivery process. Does the record reflect signs of potential fetal stress in an abnormal FHT pattern? Was the abnormality slight, moderate, or severe? Was it indicative of head compression, cord compression, or compromise of the uteroplacental unit? Was the passage of meconium present in combination with abnormal FHTs? If so, at what stage of labor was it noted? Was it dark, light, thick, or thin?
- If signs of fetal stress were present, were appropriate measures taken to correct the situation, e.g., the alteration of maternal position and administration of oxygen? If an oxytocic agent was being administered, was it discontinued at that time? If the situation was not corrected, what measures were taken? Were they appropriate and accomplished in a timely fashion?
- Ideally, the labor pattern was normal, with the fetus rotating to a normal occiput anterior (OA) position and descending to a station from which delivery could easily be effected, either spontaneously or with the assistance of low forceps. However, if abnormalities are reflected by the record, do they show an abnormal presentation, persistent minor malposition, or failure to descend?

- Was there a sudden appearance of severe fetal distress? If there was a need for immediate delivery, was it effected by the most expeditious method available to the individual physician with the available personnel and facilities? Were the facilities adequate? Was the method, considering the presenting circumstances, the one that was the most likely to be the least traumatic for the mother and infant?
- If a claim concerns maternal mortality or morbidity, does a sequential pattern emerge from the pertinent intrapartum and postpartum records that reveals the onset of the problem and the potential etiology?
- For claims involving stillbirth or neonatal mortality or morbidity, was the placenta sent to surgical pathology for diagnosis of potential, contributory abnormalities?
- If the fetus was stillborn or died in the neonatal period, was an autopsy performed to rule out any potential genetic or congenital factors that might have been present? If an autopsy was requested and permission denied by the parents, a plaintiff's subsequent claim will be more difficult to pursue when the physician is not allowed to rule out all possible etiologic factors.
- What was the level of expertise of the person who performed the pathologic examination of the placenta or who did the neonatal autopsy? The surgical pathologist who has not examined a large number of normal placentas may not easily identify one that is abnormal. Likewise, the physician performing a neonatal autopsy may not recognize subtle abnormalities if he does not have special knowledge and skills in neuropathology.

Neonatal and Pediatric Records

Claims often involve infants who survive and subsequently develop symptoms of a central nervous system disorder. In such instances, all data regarding the infant from the moment of delivery until the date of dismissal—the neonatal record—plus all pediatric records to date should be closely examined.

- In the neonatal record, special attention should be given to the initial Apgar score, resuscitation methods needed, physical examination, measurements, appearance, vital signs, and neurologic response. When was the onset of the problem noted? What attempts were made to diagnose the etiology of the problem? What treatment was initiated to correct the problem or to stabilize the infant?

Laboratory, radiology, and/or pathology data are valuable in determining which factors were present prior to the onset of labor, during the course of labor, during the actual delivery, or in the neonatal period. In addition, nurses' notes often describe dysmorphic features or abnormalities in appearance that may not have been noted at the time of the initial examination.

The most important thought to keep in mind when evaluating neonatal records is that neonatal depression and central nervous system dysfunction are not necessarily synonymous with an intrapartum insult that could have been avoided. A thorough analysis explores the many other factors that can cause the fetus to respond poorly during the birth process and subsequently to react poorly to the extrauterine environment.

Examining all pediatric records involving the child to date often reveals clues to alternate potential etiologies for the child's injury. These records often contain the diagnosis that the child's problem is secondary to an intrapartum, perinatal event, e.g., "perinatal hypoxia," "neonatal hypoxic-ischemic encephalopathy," "asphyxia neonatorum," or "birth trauma." When such a diagnosis is based solely on the history given by the parents, and when the authenticity of the diagnosis is not supported by the actual neonatal record, the defense should request a complete medical and genetic evaluation of the child.

Alternate Hypothesis

An alternate hypothesis is a defined etiology for an injury, projected by the defense, which differs from that alleged by the plaintiff. Conclusions of medical causation are too often based on assumptions made by observing a specific event which became manifest in a short period of time when, in fact, predisposing factors may have led to the complication or injury. In addition, the true etiology of a specific injury is not always clear-cut and may be quite different from that alleged by the plaintiff.

Therefore, a thorough claims analysis should be made in the same manner used by a physician to manage a patient with an individual complaint—with the knowledge that appropriate treatment cannot be initiated until a differential diagnosis has been considered. The analyst must examine the total medical record in the same way that an expert forensic pathologist would perform an autopsy, understanding that the gross examination often tells only part of the story, that portion of the diagnosis that could be reached strictly by assumption. A microscopic examination, therefore, is absolutuely essential and, more often than not, reveals that the diagnosis made by assumption is not certain or even probable. The legal discovery process may reveal other important factors that may have played a role in the alleged injury, none of which may have been iatrogenic.

> The etiology of a newborn's neonatal depression, hypotonia, onset of seizures, and subsequent neurologic injury was assumed to be secondary to a breech presentation and prolapse of the umbilical cord prior to delivery. During the course of litigation, the examining medical expert for the defense discovered that the child's neurologic injury was, in fact, secondary to a hereditary metabolic disease. This discovery was important not only to the outcome of the litigation, but also for the parents who could have unwittingly repeated the tragedy by having another child.

All potential etiologic possibilities should be considered and further explored by the defense. As illustrated, one of these possibilities may later be found to be the truth rather than simply an alternate hypothesis.

Claim Summary

In summarizing a claim, the analyst must remember that the plaintiff bears the burden of proof. The plaintiff must show:

1. that an injury occurred;
2. that a standard of care exists for the particular procedure or practice;
3. that the defendant-doctor deviated from this standard; and
4. that the specific deviation caused the injury.

The terms *injury, deviation,* and *causation* are not synonymous. Because an injury occurred does not equate with the assumption that there was a deviation from the medical standard. Neither does the fact that a deviation from the standard occurred equate with the assumption that said deviation *caused* the alleged injury.

The thorough claims analysis speaks to all components that are necessary for the plaintiff to receive a valid recovery or award. Conclusions must never be drawn by assumption. Rather, they must be based on an honest evaluation of the factual, historical data as reflected by the available records.

Supporting Scientific Data

Defense counsel must understand the nature of the claim he is defending. The claims analyst provides appropriate medical data from the scientific literature to establish a basis for the available facts pertinent to the specific claim. When proposing an alternate hypothesis, the analyst should make available the scientific data that support such a possibility.

Trial Format

If the case goes to trial, the claims analyst organizes the information gained during discovery with previous findings to produce a medical chronology, to detail allegations and issues, and to list points to establish.

Medical Chronology

The original medical chronology is updated to include additional records received during the discovery period. To facilitate identification of a specific record during the trial, each notation in the medical chronology is numbered to correspond with the same number in the actual medical record.

Allegations and Issues

Each case has unique allegations and issues that are listed separately. For every allegation and issue, the data to be presented during the course of the trial are chronologically detailed. These allegations and issues should be extrapolated from:

1. actual medical records;
2. hospital policy and national standards;
3. scientific data and literature admitted into evidence;
4. depositions of plaintiffs;
5. depositions of defendants;

6. depositions of all parties involved in the trial matter, including nurses, treating and consulting physicians, and family members planning to testify;
7. letters of opinion and depositions of all experts for plaintiffs and defendants; and
8. depositions and trial testimony of all experts which have been given in prior cases and are relevant to the present case for impeachment purposes.

Points to Establish

Specific medical-legal points that the defense should establish by the end of the trial should be listed. A plan by which each point can be effected through the individual witnesses should be detailed.

Conclusion

When the claims analysis is made before the lawsuit is filed, this early intervention allows both the insurance company and the defense counsel to be cognizant of the medical facts as they initially appear, to be aware of the strong as well as the weak points of the case, and to be knowledgeable in all areas of potential defense. If the case is filed, the initial analysis provides the defense guidance in exploring all the possibilities during the discovery period.

By the time depositions are taken in a case, the plaintiff's attorney has already concluded that his client is gravely injured and that the treating physician should or could have prevented the injury. He has gathered his medical experts who will testify that there is, in fact, injury and that the medical records reflect deviations from the medical standard. There are, of course, often gray areas concerning possible medical deviation from the standard, and resultant causation for the injury may be a great deal less than probable or certain. By the time of deposition, however, plaintiff's counsel has already molded all of the gray areas into a picture that is projected as *plaintiff clear*—not only black and white, but vividly and dramatically touched with the mental imagery of Technicolor.

Although the plaintiff bears the burden of proof in a lawsuit, defense counsel may be medically unknowledgeable in regard to the alleged injury, unaware that treatment may have involved medical judgment versus negligence, unaware that circumstances surrounding the occurrence precluded the optimal result, or, most importantly, unaware that the etiology of the alleged injury may have been other than that projected by the plaintiff's counsel. In such a case, the burden of proof shifts, forcing the defense to prove that the plaintiff is incorrect in her assumptions.

The old cliche that the best defense is a good offense is certainly applicable. Early intervention and a thorough claims analysis, offering alternate hypotheses and supportive scientific data for exploration, allow the insurance company and defense counsel to be knowledgeable and prepared. The defendant-doctor is not immediately forced to bear the burden of assumption, and the burden of proof then rests, as it should, with the plaintiff.

Chapter 16

The Hospital and the Physician, Partners in Loss Prevention

Charles M. Jacobs and Daniel K. Roberts

As the number of medical malpractice claims and the size of awards have grown, the interpretation of hospital and physician liability has changed radically. Understandably, changes in the malpractice liability environment have demanded reevaluation and modification of the physician-hospital relationship. Physicians have, however, viewed these modifications as offensive because they seem to equate with increased scrutiny of the practice of medicine by hospital boards of trustees, administrators, and other laymen. These modifications are perceived as placing in the hands of administrators and regulators critical clinical decisions about which patients are admitted, what series of tests are allowed, what kinds of operative procedures can be done and who can do them, how long the patient can stay in the hospital, and what kind of follow-up documentation must appear on the medical charts. These restrictions generally stem from the hospital medical staff's own bylaws, rules, and regulations that have been modified in recent years to reflect statutory, regulatory, legal, and other external pressures, many of which relate to issues of liability for health care services.

We shall first examine the basis for the changing liability climate and its influence on both medical practice and the hospital-physician relationship. Secondly, we shall point out how mutual self-interest requires active participation in risk management and loss prevention programs by the physician, the hospital administration, and the hospital's governing board.

The Basis of Hospital Liability

Until recently, there were three basic ways in which a hospital could be found liable for patient injury.

1. Environmental hazards—for example, patient injuries resulting from falling on wet floors, equipment malfunction, etc.
2. Respondeat superior—a legal concept assigning liability to the employer for employee actions undertaken on the job. For example, the hospital would be liable if a patient was injured by falling out of bed after a nurse failed to raise the bed rails as required or if a patient reacted to a unit of blood inappropriately labeled by a blood bank technician.
3. Apparent agency—another legal concept that assumes the patient relied on the hospital to act as an agent in securing certain medical services. For example, generally the pathologist, emergency room physician, anesthesiologist, or radiologist is selected by the hospital, not by the patient. If one of these hospital-based physicians negligently injures the patient, the hospital may be found liable for the physician's negligence because of the apparent agency relationship.

The courts recently embraced the theory of corporate liability to cover the acts of independent practitioners, thereby rapidly increasing the hospital's and the medical staff's exposure to loss. Traditionally, hospitals claimed no corporate responsibility for the acts of physicians independently retained by the patient. When a patient sued a hospital for injury due to physician negligence, the hospital replied that the direct relationship was between patient and private physician, not between patient and hospital. Put simply, the hospital maintained no responsibility for the acts of independent contractors. A growing body of case law rejects this traditional defense and extends corporate liability to the hospital, under certain conditions. We shall examine some of the reasons for the reinterpretation.

Technology Explosion

As medical technology mushroomed and as more people gained access to increasingly complex, hospital-oriented medical care, society began to reassess its relationship with health care providers. The era in which the family physician's black bag carried the preponderance of medical technology has disappeared forever. The average person, overwhelmed by the complexity of the health care system, demanded assurance that someone take responsibility for managing the technology and insuring its safety. As in other sectors, rapid technological change led to legal change, as the following example illustrates.

Common law has long required that the injured party demonstrate a direct relationship with the alleged cause of the injury. Here is a simple example. A customer in a small Mom and Pop corner grocery store picks up a bottle of soda pop. On the way to the checkout counter the improperly manufactured bottle explodes, blinding the man. Who is liable for this injury? The owners of the Mom and Pop grocery store or the manufacturer and bottler of the soft drink? Intuition would suggest the bottler, and today's courts would agree. Traditionally, however, common law would have disagreed, finding that no direct relationship existed between the bottler and the customer.

Why did society and eventually the law come to extend liability even where no direct relationship existed between the injured person and the alleged cause? The answer lies in the nature of technology. Soft drink bottling, for example, involves an understanding of the tensile strength of glass, properties of gaseous mixtures, and other complex concepts. Clearly this technology is beyond the comprehension of the average grocery store proprietor or customer. Also, the effects of technology are not localized near the point of production but rather may be distributed widely and may involve persons all over the country. Society came to expect those who operate and benefit most directly from the use of technology to guarantee its safety. The courts shifted their focus because the purpose of legal liability is twofold. First, the injured party must be indemnified. But from a broader perspective, the purpose of liability is deterrence. Therefore, the party who can act on or respond to information or to the fear of financial penalty became the focus of liability.

In our example, the soft drink bottler, not the grocer, has the ability to modify the technology to prevent similar injuries by exploding bottles. Society requires the bottler, as keeper of the technology, to prevent injury and indemnify injurious results from negligence.

Changes in Physician and Hospital Liability

How do these changes in the concepts of liability and responsibility for technology specifically relate to physicians and hospitals? Before we can answer, we must first ask, what exactly are hospitals? Although hospitals differ widely, some common essential characteristics exist. Hospitals are legal entities with a board of trustees, an organized medical staff, full-time registered nurse coverage, full-time administration, and a variety of technical and support personnel. Hospitals function to provide an environment in which the physician-patient interchange can take place. Hospitals cannot, by law, practice medicine. Therefore, hospitals need physicians and, given the complexity of modern medicine, physicians need hospitals to provide and organize the technology.

Who then, in the modern health care system, is responsible for gathering and using information to prevent patient injury in the hospital setting? Society's answer in many circumstances is the hospital.

Hospital care involves too many people and too much technology to reasonably place the full burden of deterrence on the patient's private physician. But, hospitals have resisted this shift in legal liability to the institution.

Hospitals first argued immunity from malpractice on the grounds that it was inappropriate to sue charitable organizations, thereby diverting funds from the social welfare. This defense crumbled because, since the 1960s, hospital funds have come mainly from patient billings—paid by private insurers or government entities—and not from charitable contributions.

Second, facilities named in physician malpractice suits attacked the applicability of the legal basis of negligence. To prove the hospital negligent, the plaintiff must establish:

1. that a duty was owed the patient by the facility;
2. that the hospital breached this duty;
3. that measurable harm occurred to the patient; and
4. that the breach of duty was causally related to the measurable injury.

Hospitals traditionally argued that in the case of patients treated by private physicians, the hospital had no duty to the patient. The courts, in landmark decisions, asserted that a hospital's duty could be extended to controlling the independent individual physician's actions when those had a propensity to cause patient harm.

The *Darling* Case

Darling v. Charleston Community Memorial Hospital followed from a general practitioner treating a patient for a broken leg.[1] The physician failed to respond to symptoms indicating that the cast was too tight during the two weeks the patient was hospitalized. No consultation was requested. The patient subsequently lost his leg to amputation secondary to the complications. The physician settled out of court and the hospital was also found liable in the landmark decision. The physician was not an employee and, therefore, the principle of respondeat superior did not apply.

In its defense the hospital contended that

> only an individual properly educated and licensed, and not a corporation, may practice medicine . . . accordingly a hospital with respect to actual medical care of a professional nature is to use reasonable care in selecting medical doctors. When such in the selection of the staff is accomplished, and nothing indicates that a physician so selected is incompetent or that such incompetence should have been discovered, more cannot be expected from the hospital administration [p. 254].

The Illinois Supreme Court affirmed the jury verdict against the hospital:

> 'The conception that the hospital does not undertake to treat the patient, does not undertake to act through its doctors and nurses but undertakes instead simply to procure them to act upon their own responsibility no longer reflects the facts . . . . Certainly the person who avails himself of "hospital facilities" expects that the hospital will attempt to cure him, not that its nurses or other employees will act on their own responsibilities. *Bing v. Thunig (N.Y. 1957).*' The Standards for Hospital Accreditation, the state licensing regulations and the defendant's bylaws demonstrate that the medical profession and other responsible authorities regard it as both desirable and reasonable that a hospital assume certain responsibilities for the care of the patient . . . . As to consultation, there is no dispute that the hospital failed to review Dr. Alexander's work or require a consultation. The only issue is whether its failure to do so was negligence. On the evidence before it the jury could reasonably have found that it was [pp. 255–256].

This case awakened hospital administrators and their counsels all over the country. In essence it said that hospitals were liable not on just what they knew about a physician but for what they should have known in order to fulfill their duty to assure proper treatment.

The *Darling* case has been followed or paralleled in a growing number of cases which generally follow the view expressed in *Fiorentino v. Wegner.*[2]

> Where there is no vicarious liability, the plaintiff must establish that the hospital . . . was guilty of malpractice or other tort concurring in causing the harm . . . . [A] hospital will not be held liable for an act of malpractice performed by an independently retained healer, unless it had reason to know that the act of malpractice would take place [p. 299].

Two other cases that paralleled the *Darling* decision are worthy of brief mention.

In *Joiner v. Mitchell County Hospital Authority,* an emergency room physician misdiagnosed a myocardial infarction and sent the patient home.[3] Shortly afterward, the patient was dead on arrival in the emergence room. The patient's widow filed against the physician and hospital. She claimed the hospital did not adequately evaluate the professional qualifications of the physician and negligently appointed him to the staff. The hospital countered that it was not liable because the physician was licensed by the state of Georgia and because the screening of physician applicants was conducted by the medical staff. The Supreme Court of Georgia upheld the plaintiff's verdict, saying, in essence:

1. the cause of action was valid not on respondeat superior, but based on the hospital's independent duty to assure appropriate care to the patient;
2. the hospital through its board has the power to screen physician applicants and limit privileges; and
3. when making credentials recommendations, the medical staff members act as agents of the hospital.

In *Purcell v. Zimbelman,* the verdict resulted in monies paid by Tucson General Hospital.[4] A general surgeon intraoperatively misdiagnosed a case of diverticulitis as cancer without requesting a frozen section which was available. As a result of this misdiagnosis, a major cancer procedure was inappropriately decided upon and accomplished, resulting in major injury to the patient. During the trial, it was discovered that two similar malpractice suits involving performance of the same procedure at the same hospital had previously occurred. The hospital argued that since the two previous cases had been reviewed with no action by a committee in the hospital's department of surgery who were independent doctors on the staff, the hospital was not liable for inaction. In essence, the Arizona court said:

1. the department of surgery was acting on behalf of the hospital and their negligence of inaction is the hospital's negligence;
2. the hospital was negligent in its failure to assure its duty to a patient was properly performed; and
3. the prior malpractice cases put the hospital on notice and it *should have known* of the questionable competence of the physician.

Gonzales v. Nork

The judge's well-reasoned memorandum in *Gonzales v. Nork and Mercy Hospital,* a 1973 California case, clearly illustrates the legal basis of the hospital's duty to patients and its liability for negligence in failing to protect its patients from injury by independent practitioners.[5] Dr. Nork, an orthopedic surgeon, performed laminectomies on patients at Mercy and other area hospitals for a nine-year period. The results were often poor. Prior to Gonzales, on whom Nork operated in 1967, two other suits were brought against Dr. Nork. Mercy Hospital had no knowledge of this record until it learned in 1970 that Dr. Nork's malpractice insurance had been canceled. At that time, the hospital acted swiftly to limit Dr. Nork's activities.

The question before the court was whether Mercy Hospital had failed its duty to the patient, Mr. Gonzales, by not acting sooner, and thereby failing to protect him from Dr. Nork's injurious actions. Mercy Hospital's defenses were:

1. it owed no duty to the patient for treatment provided by independent medical staff members—the independent contractor theory;
2. even if it had a duty, accreditation from the Joint Commission on Accreditation of Hospitals (JCAH) demonstrated that the duty was fulfilled; and
3. JCAH and California's law required delegation of responsibility for supervising medical care to the organized medical staff.

The court ruled for the patient and against the hospital. First the court maintained that the hospital owed a duty to the patient.

> The hospital by virtue of its custody of the patient, owes him a duty . . . to protect him from acts of malpractice by his independently retained physician . . . if the hospital knows, or has reason to know, or should have known that such acts were likely to occur [pp. 153–154].

The court also rejected the defense that JCAH accreditation met this obligation.

> Mercy Hospital contends that because it complied with (JCAH) standards, it cannot be held negligent. It has not argued that hospitals have the 'privilege, which is usually emphatically denied to other groups, of setting their own standards of conduct, merely by adopting their own practices.' Nor would such an argument prevail here, because, as will be shown hereafter, we are dealing with problems in the area of medical science. It is no more

a matter of medical science to require a hospital to tally up a doctor's lapses
than it is to require a nurse to count sponges . . . [pp. 166–167].

In addition, the court noted, "The testimony . . . shows that the JCAH
standards being followed by Mercy Hospital at the time of Gonzales'
surgery were deficient . . ." (p. 182). Finally, although the hospital did
have an organized medical staff, as required by law and JCAH, the
court indicated, "This does not immunize it from liability, because the
medical staff acts for the hospital in discharge of the hospital's responsibilities to protect its patients" (p. 164).

An ongoing body of case law reinforces the principles set forth in
the *Nork* case. As a result, hospitals clearly have a legal as well as a
moral obligation to implement systems for protecting patients. How
does a hospital discharge this obligation?

Participation in Loss Prevention

Hospitals exist primarily so that independent physicians can treat
their acutely ill patients. Ultimate or fiduciary responsibility for the
hospital rests with its board of trustees. The board of trustees, however,
by law, must delegate to an organized medical staff the right to provide
medical services. Individual physicians share this right only by becoming members of the staff.

The hospital, through the board of trustees, has the duty to acquire
and use information to prevent patient harm. Although these functions
are medicoadministrative rather than clinical, the board of trustees
usually delegates to the medical staff such peer review functions as
evaluating and monitoring care, credentialing, and participating in loss
prevention activities.

The individual medical staff member remains responsible and legally
liable for clinical failures due to performance below the standard of
care. The hospital, however, and even the entire medical staff may be
liable for injuries that probably would not have occurred if the medicoadministrative system had not failed. Specifically, the hospital and
potentially the entire staff are at risk if:

1. a failure to acquire and/or use knowledge is demonstrated; and
2. a responsible attempt to acquire and use the information could
   have prevented the injury.

For example, in the Wisconsin case *Johnson v. Misericordia Community Hospital*, the hospital was found liable for not deterring the

injury to a patient by a private physician, Dr. Salinsky.[6] The court stated: "Johnson *was only obliged to prove that Misericordia did not make a reasonable effort to determine whether Salinsky was qualified to perform orthopedic surgery*" (p. 172). In *Corleto v. Shore Memorial Hospital*, the trial court ruled that the patient alleging injury could sue the entire medical staff or each of the 141 members individually.[7] The plaintiff argued that since the entire hospital medical staff voted on membership issues, they were liable for the injury allegedly due to the failure of the credentialing system.

Conclusion

In conclusion, the crucial points to carry away from this chapter are:

1. hospitals may be liable for patient injuries by private physicians;
2. if directly or through the medicoadministrative functions delegated to the medical staff, the hospital should have known that injury was likely to occur, then negligence may be attributed; and
3. the hospital must be able to demonstrate that reasonable systems, implemented in good faith, exist for reviewing patient care and for granting and reassessing staff membership and clinical privileges.

Understanding these points should encourage medical practitioners to support appropriate policies and actions that contribute to a comprehensive loss prevention program, thereby helping not only hospitals and physicians but ultimately patients as well.

References

1. *Darling v. Charleston Community Memorial Hospital,* 211 NE2d 253, 1965.
2. *Fiorentino v. Wenger,* 227 NE2d 296, 1967.
3. *Joiner v. Mitchell County Hospital Authority,* 189 SE2d 412, 1972.
4. *Purcell v. Zimbelman,* 500 P2d 335, 1972.
5. *Gonzales v. Nork and Mercy Hospital,* Superior Court of California, Sacramento County: No. 225866, 1973.
6. *Johnson v. Misericordia Community Hospital,* 301 NW2d 156, 1981.
7. *Corleto v. Shore Memorial Hospital,* 350 A2d 534, 1975.

Chapter 17

Risk Management and Loss Prevention in the Hospital

Charles M. Jacobs and Daniel K. Roberts

Traditionally, a hospital's risk management program encompasses those organizational components and functions that are associated with the acquisition and maintenance of insurance coverage and with internal claims administration and management. In today's litigation-prone environment, however, such a narrowly defined risk management program will provide the institution with equally narrow and inadequate protection from loss related to alleged patient injury. A comprehensive risk management program must include, in addition to the insurance and claims management functions, loss prevention systems and intervention strategies for loss reduction.

Put simply, the difference between the traditional system and that which is appropriate for the modern hospital is the difference between a *reactive* and a *proactive* approach to risk. With million-dollar-plus malpractice awards now part of hospital reality, facilities can no longer afford to wait for claims to be filed before action commences. Hospitals must implement *loss prevention* systems to detect and correct situations that may generate potentially compensable events (PCEs). In addition, when a patient injury occurs, the facility must initiate *loss reduction* strategies, make timely approaches to the patient, as well as document and develop alternative hypotheses with the objective of minimizing the potential financial loss to the institution.

Although risk management in the broadest sense includes insuring against, preventing, and reducing loss from all forms of liability, we focus on the major source of loss—medical malpractice. Therefore, in this overview of the essentials of comprehensive risk management as well as loss prevention and reduction, we emphasize the role of the physician's clinical expertise.

Components of a Risk Management Program

A comprehensive risk management program entails four primary functions: (1) risk or exposure identification; (2) risk-related data analysis; (3) risk treatment and insurance; and (4) risk management program evaluation.

Risk or Exposure Identification

Risk or exposure identification requires a systematic means of detecting potential losses, as well as patterns of events or behavior related to the potential for loss. To accomplish this task requires a thorough understanding of hospital operations, existing sources of data for risk identification and monitoring, and potential sources of data relevant to risk management functions.

A comprehensive risk management program begins with an inventory of hospital organizational components, personnel, and data systems. This inventory provides the basis for an analysis of the hospital's present risk management and loss prevention situation (see Table 1).

Table 1

Sample Components for a Hospital Risk Management Inventory

Medical Staff
1. Size and professional characteristics;
2. Open or closed staff status;
3. Controls on membership, the granting of clinical privileges, and reappointment;
4. Quality review and control mechanisms;
5. Bylaws, structure, and other mechanisms for self-governing.

Nursing Staff
1. Size and professional characteristics (RN/LPN mix, primary nursing, etc.);
2. Organization;

Table 1

(Continued)

Nursing Staff (Continued)

3. Supply and demand (use of pools, etc.);
4. Selection, credentialing, and retention;
5. Quality assurance and control;
6. In-service training and educational programs.

Other Personnel

1. Categories and numbers;
2. Credentialing, privileging, and review mechanisms;
3. Supply and demand, retention, and turnover;
4. In-service training and educational programs.

Patient Care Policies and Processes

1. Specifications for clinical supervision of patient care units and services;
2. Special supervision, credentialing, mandatory consultation requirements, or restriction of personnel dealing with special equipment, critical care patients, etc.;
3. Existence of patient care procedures specified in procedural manuals, including delineation of documentation requirements;
4. Procedures for handling STAT orders, lab panic values, etc.

Equipment and Supplies

1. Existence of a mechanism for clinical input on the selection of equipment and supplies;
2. Existence of a mechanism for recording and monitoring, over time, incidents related to equipment and supply failures and for using this information in the purchasing process;
3. Existence of an ongoing safety and maintenance program;
4. Existence of a program for orienting relevant personnel to the use and care of new equipment.

Claims Experience

1. Historical claims experience, both lawsuits and claims made in writing by patients' attorneys.

Incidence Reports and Patient Complaints

1. Incident reports;
2. Patient complaints documented by patient representatives, advocates, or other personnel;
3. Patient satisfaction questionnaires administered by the hospital or component services.

Logs or Other Hospital Documentation

1. Pharmacy or blood bank monitoring data, e.g., inappropriate ordering or reactions;
2. Surgery logs, etc.

186 CONFRONTING THE MALPRACTICE CRISIS

The data compiled as part of the risk identification process should present a picture of the hospital, its resources, and its risk and loss history. Ideally, analysis of the initial data available should identify:

1. patterns of incidences and loss;
2. level of estimated comprehensiveness of incident reporting, i.e., claims initially documented by incident reports;
3. patterns of reporting by professional category, service, type of event, etc.;
4. incentives and disincentives to early identification of potentially compensable events;
5. timeliness of intervention and documentation, including the effect on the eventual outcome of the potentially compensable event; and
6. appropriateness of the use of risk-related data, i.e., feedback to hospital functions and staff.

In most hospitals, however, existing risk identification systems will pick up only sixty percent of the potentially compensable events. In fact, in many instances, the facility's first awareness of a problem involving patient injury from a clinical act of omission or commission is receipt of the summons. Clearly, traditional incident-reporting systems miss a large portion of potentially compensable events. An adequate risk identification system should identify events, particularly untoward clinical events, ideally during the hospital stay but certainly no later than at discharge. Timely identification of individual events allows:

1. intervention with the patient and the family to ameliorate problems;
2. coordination to assure accuracy, completeness, and quality of all medicolegal documentation; and
3. development of alternate clinical hypotheses and their documentation while evidence and memories are still fresh.

An example of a useful mechanism for timely identification of untoward clinical events is the Clinical Occurrence Screening System, developed by InterQual as a result of the California Medical Insurance Feasibility Study.[1] This system relies upon concurrent screening for objective evidence of untoward clinical events primarily documented in the medical record. The objective of the Clinical Occurrence Screening System is to identify potentially compensable events for further analysis and/or action as necessary. Such an early warning system not only increases the timely identification of and intervention in individual cases, but also provides an essential data base for risk analysis.

Risk-Related Data Analysis

Once systems and data sources for identifying loss possibilities are in place, the second phase in the risk management process, risk analysis, begins. The general objective of risk analysis is to determine which exposures are significant enough to manage and which ones can be safely ignored. Specific objectives are to determine:

1. the probable frequency of occurrence of loss;
2. the probable severity of loss;
3. the possible severity of loss; and
4. the potential effects that any loss would have on the organization from both a financial and operational perspective.

Particularly because of the paucity of data about the true incidence rate of potentially compensable events, estimation of the *probable frequency of occurrence of loss* is generally based on historic analysis of claims. Implementation of a risk identification system valuably augments this claims-based analysis by providing solid data on which to base estimates of the underlying risk or incidence of untoward clinical events that have the potential to generate claims and losses. Until the individual hospital generates sufficient data for aggregation and analysis, the results of the California Medical Insurance Feasibility Study may be used as a benchmark.* In addition, hospital-specific claims data may be augmented with the National Association of Insurance Commissioners' study,† which is a detailed nationwide analysis of the malpractice claims that were closed between 1975 and 1978.[2]

The *probable severity of loss* represents an estimate of the most likely dollar value of the loss the hospital would sustain during a given time period, assuming normal operations.

The *possible severity of loss* assumes the worst case and attempts to identify the maximum possible exposure to financial loss.

---

* See Appendix B for a summary of the results of the California Medical Insurance Feasibility Study.

† See Appendix A for a summary of the results of the National Association of Insurance Commissioners' Study.

Finally, the *potential effects* on the institution of sustaining either the probable loss or the maximum possible loss must be considered. These include direct, indirect, and moral costs. Direct costs are those that accrue from actual dollar loss and its impact on the institution's continued viability. Indirect effects influence the institution's ability to attract patients, physicians, and personnel. The moral costs that result when a healing institution causes patient injury or death must also be evaluated.

The direct, indirect, and moral costs that could be associated with either the probable or the maximum possible loss form one-half of a theoretical cost-benefit analysis. This analysis measures the *cost* of insurance or of improving a procedure, equipment, staffing level, or other preventive measure relative to the *benefit* associated with expected reduction of costs due to the probable or possible loss. The benefit may be a reduction of moral costs rather than direct dollar savings and may greatly alter the balance of this equation.

This type of loss estimation and cost-benefit risk analysis is useful in separating types of events and in setting priorities for intervention. Estimating the probability that different potentially compensable events will occur, estimating the expected amount of compensation, estimating the probability that loss prevention activities will succeed, and estimating the cost of intervention are admittedly difficult. Nevertheless, the risk analysis approach structures the hospital's consideration of a complex situation.

Problems and patterns identified by a risk identification system, incidence reports, and other information sources may at least be categorized using a risk analysis matrix (see Table 2). Identifying which cell on the matrix a particular problem falls into can help to set risk management program priorities and objectives. For example, problems in cell 2 clearly should be addressed, while problems in cell 13 usually would not be worth the effort or expense. Trade-offs between addressing problems in cells 5 and 7, however, may need to be negotiated within the organization.

Risk Treatment and Insurance

Once the risk has been identified and assessed, there are two approaches to risk treatment: risk control techniques (loss prevention and loss reduction); and risk financing (risk retention or transfer by insurance or other means).

Table 2

Risk Analysis Matrix

1	2	3	4
Probability of Event: High Probable $ Loss: High Probability Preventable: High Cost of Prevention: High	Probability of Event: High Probable $ Loss: High Probability Preventable: High Cost of Prevention: Low	Probability of Event: High Probable $ Loss: High Probability Preventable: High Cost of Prevention: Low	Probability of Event: High Probable $ Loss: Low Probability Preventable: High Cost of Prevention: High

5	6	7	8
Probability of Event: Low Probable $ Loss: High Probability Preventable: High Cost of Prevention: High	Probability of Event: Low Probable $ Loss: High Probability Preventable: High Cost of Prevention: High	Probability of Event: Low Probable $ Loss: High Probability Preventable: High Cost of Prevention: Low	Probability of Event: High Probable $ Loss: Low Probability Preventable: Low Cost of Prevention: High

9	10	11	12
Probability of Event: Low Probable $ Loss: High Probability Preventable: Low Cost of Prevention: Low	Probability of Event: Low Probable $ Loss: High Probability Preventable: Low Cost of Prevention: Low	Probability of Event: High Probable $ Loss: High Probability Preventable: Low Cost of Prevention: Low	Probability of Event: Low Probable $ Loss: Low Probability Preventable: High Cost of Prevention: High

13	14	15	16
Probability of Event: Low Probable $ Loss: Low Probability Preventable: Low Cost of Prevention: High	Probability of Event: Low Probable $ Loss: Low Probability Preventable: Low Cost of Prevention: High	Probability of Event: Low Probable $ Loss: High Probability Preventable: High Cost of Prevention: Low	Probability of Event: Low Probable $ Loss: Low Probability Preventable: High Cost of Prevention: Low

Risk control techniques are attempts to achieve better control over the loss-producing activities themselves. Such control can be accomplished by:

1. Loss prevention—reducing the frequency of loss-producing events.*

   Example: Limiting the surgical privileges of a physician after the hospital's risk identification system *and* peer review indicate an exceptionally high rate of unplanned patient returns to the operating room due to inadequate performance of the initial procedure.

   Example: Carpeting of all floors may eliminate falls that result from slippery wet tile or other smooth surface floors.

   Example: An instrument count in surgical operating rooms prevents surgical instruments from being left inside patients.

2. Loss reduction—decreasing potential severity of loss exposures.

   Example: A code blue or STAT team minimizes loss by responding to cardiac or respiratory distressed patients.

   Example: A sprinkler system may retard the spread of fire until it is extinguished, decreasing injuries to nonambulatory patients.

Physician involvement constitutes an integral part of both loss prevention and loss reduction activities related to clinical events. The physician must be involved in risk control by reviewing individual cases that fall through the hospital's risk identification system, by providing peer review mechanisms when possible patterns of untoward events are identified, by activating credentialing, privileging, and other medical staff interventions as appropriate, and by providing alternate clinical hypotheses for claims management.

Risk financing is another technique used to manage and pay for losses. Risk retention and risk transfer are the two major subcategories.

1. Risk retention or assumption occurs when a hospital assumes the financial burden of certain risk exposures rather than purchasing insurance coverage. Risk retention may not be deliberate, as hap-

---

* Loss prevention also may be achieved by a claims management program resulting in a well-prepared defense to claims thereby reducing or controlling the amount of dollar loss or settlement.

pens when the hospital fails to recognize the existence of certain risks. On the other hand, it may be the result of careful deliberation, as when a hospital establishes a self-insurance program. Common forms of risk retention are:

- unfunded self-insurance—funding for the cost of loss exposures that is not provided in advance;
- funded self-insurance—funding provided in advance to cover the cost of anticipated loss exposures;
- pooled self-insurance—funding to cover anticipated losses based on the concept of several hospitals forming a joint self-insurance venture;
- a single-owner or multi-owner captive insurance company— organized under the state or a foreign government; and
- fronting arrangements—when the hospital purchases an insurance contract with the agreement to participate in the risk through a hospital self-insurance mechanism, thus transferring a portion of the risk back to the hospital.

The high cost of commercial liability insurance has prompted many hospitals to investigate whether risk retention is more advantageous than commercial coverage. Retention has several advantages:

- retention costs may be much less than commercial insurance;
- commercial insurance coverage is sometimes unavailable;
- retention of some risk may entice underwriters who otherwise might not wish to expose themselves to lower layers of risk to provide amounts over the hospital's retention amount; and
- it necessitates more concern by the operating managers to reduce costs.

However, despite the advantages of retention, commercial insurance coverage does provide more security since the responsibility for worrying about the financing of future losses becomes the insurance carrier's job. A hospital contemplating substantial retention should first have a risk minimization and loss prevention program in place as well as provisions for good claims management services.

2. Risk transfer involves the assumption of risk by a third party. Commercial insurance is the most commonly used risk-financing device. The hospital transfers the financing of its loss exposures

to a third party under the terms of an insurance contract. Before this method is employed,

- the hospital's prior loss exposures should be identified, evaluated, and analyzed;
- risk control techniques should be introduced; and
- risks should be classified to determine which financing method should be used for each class.

The most common method for noninsurance risk transfer is for the party who has the exclusive legal responsibility for a particular category of loss exposure to transfer that risk to another party through a hold-harmless agreement or contract clause. In essence, such an agreement assures the first party that it will not suffer any legal harm from a specific risk it transfers to the other party.

Example: University B agrees to defend, indemnify, and keep harmless Hospital A, its agents, and its employees from any and all liability, loss, damage, and expense, including attorneys' fees, that may result from or arise out of or be in connection with the clinical affiliation programs of fourth-year student nurses.

Risk Evaluation

Evaluation is the final step in the ongoing risk management process. Regardless of the criteria used, the process of evaluative feedback closes the loop on risk management decision making. This vitally important task is not easy. Each component must be evaluated for its continuing success in meeting its objective. The following categories and questions are suggested as starting points.

Risk identification:

1. Have exposures been missed in the identification activity? If so, why?
2. What adjustments are necessary to improve this phase?
3. Are useful data being gathered?
4. Is a comprehensive data base employed and updated frequently?

Risk analysis:

1. Does the analysis process capture important quantitative data, identify patterns, and consider important qualitative issues?

2. Is an analytic process being used to make decisions on risk treatment?

Risk treatment:

1. Are risk control and risk financing methods used for each exposure type?
2. Are exposures evaluated to determine which treatment methods are appropriate?
3. Is management aware of current insurance market positions concerning availability and costs?

Organizing a Loss Prevention and Reduction Program

To conduct a malpractice loss minimization and exposure avoidance program such as we describe, a hospital must have the cooperation of its medical staff leadership. Staff physicians are codefendants in about eighty percent of all hospital malpractice actions, and the more serious malpractice actions are generally concerned with clinically related matters requiring physician analysis in the risk management process.

Essential to the risk management process are quality assurance (QA) activities, such as surgical case (tissue) review, drug and blood use monitoring, peer analysis of complications and deaths, and infection surveillance and control. First, QA activities generate data and information needed for risk management purposes. Second, in most states, such integration of QA activities gains statutory and common law immunity and nondiscovery protection for the risk management program. Nondiscovery protection attempts to assure that the QA and risk management efforts will not be subverted by allowing malpractice plaintiffs access to reviewing and monitoring material. Immunity protection attempts to assure the medical staff and hospital personnel engaged in the review function that a successful lawsuit cannot arise from the review process itself.

Medical staff members are often skeptical about hospital-based QA activities since direct benefits to individuals are sometimes difficult to demonstrate. They view loss minimization activities as more relevant to today's physician. A good risk management program protects not only the hospital but the individual physician and the patient.

In addition to the cooperation of the medical staff, a total risk management program requires hospitalwide commitment, including the board of trustees, management, employees, and contract services personnel. It must be either integrated with QA activities or complementary to these activities when total integration would be counterproductive.

Risk Manager

The loss minimization program needs an administrative focal point— a risk manager or other officer who assumes risk management functions. This individual must have the following qualifications:

1. experience in hospital operations, preferably quality assurance or administration;
2. ability to function at the level of associate or assistant administrator;
3. ability to develop and to maintain credibility with members of the medical and nursing staffs;
4. a basic understanding of medicine and the medical approach to disease and dysfunction;
5. knowledge about insurance and legal issues or capability to acquire knowledge to assure proper use of insurance and legal consultation; and,
6. aptitude in interpersonal relations and oral communications.

Although definitive guidance on the relationship of the risk manager to others in the hospital's organizational structure cannot be provided because of the vast differences in the organization of hospitals and medical staffs, there are some general rules. To function effectively, the risk manager needs broad organizational support and authority. Ideally, the president or senior vice-president should serve as the risk manager's supervisor. In addition, the specific inclusion of the risk management function in the hospital's corporate and medical staff bylaws is necessary to legitimize the responsibility of and to provide authority for the loss control function. The risk manager should participate in relevant medical staff and hospital committees. Particularly recommended is the formation of a medical staff risk identification committee or subcommittee to support the risk management efforts by providing a ready source of clinical expertise.

Board of Trustees

A risk management program cannot succeed unless the hospital's board of trustees oversees the information-gathering and use activities that relate to quality assurance and loss control. The activities at issue include:

1. systematic evaluation of practitioner performance against explicit, predetermined criteria, including criteria that specify predicted patient outcomes;
2. clinical evaluation of untoward occurrences and malpractice claims;
3. continuous monitoring of critical aspects of care, including antibiotic and drug usage, transfusion practices, review of tissue removed at surgery, and infections;
4. credentialing members of the medical and ancillary health professional staffs, using the results of performance reviews; and
5. enforcement of clinical policies and consultation requirements.

The amount of time that members of the medical staff must devote to these processes is formidable and resented by most physicians. Moreover, because the results of these processes sometimes require decisions with unpleasant consequences for peers, there is a natural tendency to avoid reaching firm conclusions. Consequently, since medical staff members avoid these essential quality assurance and loss control functions, the hospital administrator assumes a direct role in countering this avoidance phenomenon by trying to force decisions. These actions are resented, even by those staff members who recognize the need for administrative concern and the difficult decisions that must be made. Hospital administrators who become too active in this arena often place their jobs at risk.

Dealing with this organizational problem requires two strategies. The first is to have the board of trustees oversee and supervise the performance of the critical quality assurance and loss control functions through a professional affairs committee (PAC) of the board. The second is to provide administrative support to the medical staff in order to guarantee efficient use of valuable physician time. The compelling reasons for establishing an active PAC are:

1. the need for a degree of expertise at the board level concerning professional staff matters; and
2. the need for a source of authority to support demands for proper performance of quality assurance and loss control activities.

The PAC should also serve as a pressure relief valve for members of both the medical and administrative staffs. This mechanism allows the responsibility for necessary but often unpleasant disciplinary or other corrective intervention to fall on a higher authority that is less intimately involved in or dependent on the day-to-day hospital environment.

Such board supervision does not mean doing, but rather seeing that the medical staff and administration are properly managing their affairs. Those charged with governing the institution must gain some mastery over these difficult and complex issues for two reasons:

1. the provision of medical and health services is the essence of a hospital's mission; and
2. the protection of financial resources against unwarranted drain is a recognized fiduciary obligation.

Medical Staff

To avoid the fragmentation that has traditionally marked hospital quality assurance and risk management efforts, a single medical staff committee should have primary responsibility for the medical aspects of these efforts. Such a quality assurance committee (QAC) of the medical staff has a variety of functions. It determines what kind of quality assurance and loss control information should be gathered for review of medical staff activities. It coordinates the quality assurance information needs of other patient care departments and services. It reviews not only the findings of departmental patient care evaluation (audit) activities but also the reports of its subcommittees, such as:

1. a subcommittee for clinical care monitoring, e.g., blood utilization, antibiotic use, tissue review, infection surveillance;
2. a subcommittee for utilization review, e.g., admissions, lengths of stay, use of ancillary services;
3. a subcommittee for occurrence and claims analysis; and
4. a subcommittee for coordinating clinical service evaluation activities.

The QAC coordinates analysis of findings, recommendations, and actions. These recommendations are communicated to the medical executive committee, to other medical staff members, to other components responsible for using information, to the board of trustees through its PAC, and to hospital management, including the risk manager. The information collected by this integrated staffwide approach to quality assurance provides an important data base for loss prevention and loss reduction program decision making.

Summary

Risk management and loss prevention activities are essential components in a hospital's total management, information, and quality assurance programs. They are mandated by fiduciary obligations to preserve assets, by ethical obligations to prevent avoidable harm, and by professional obligations to provide the best possible care to patients. This chapter has outlined the components and organizational strategies required for meaningful risk management and loss prevention in the hospital.

References

1. Mills, DH, ed. Report on the medical insurance feasibility study. San Francisco: California Medical Association, 1977.
2. Sowka, MP, ed. Malpractice claims: final compilation: medical malpractice closed claims, 1975–1978. Brookfield, WI: National Association of Insurance Commissioners, 1980.

Entering the Future

The technological explosion has given physicians the opportunity to probe deeper, detect sooner, and intervene more successfully. However, these advances have fostered unrealistic expectations of doctors and their science, and nowhere has this been more evident than in the specialty of obstetrics and gynecology. We explore the areas within this specialty that are on the leading edge of the technological explosion. Entering the future of medical practice is a challenging prospect, but one that must be tempered by the legal lessons of the past and the present.

Chapter 18

Legal Implications of Diagnostic Radiology and Ultrasound in Obstetrics and Gynecology

John A. Anderson

Diagnostic Radiology and Nuclear Medicine

Modern medicine is no longer conducted through a series of encounters between a single physician and his patient. More and more people and devices have been interposed between this basic duo as medical science attempts to refine diagnoses and improve therapeutic outcomes. With this growth in complexity has come a concomitant alteration in the types and variety of personal injury lawsuits that are based on negligence, product liability, and strict liability in tort. New legal concepts such as wrongful life, inappropriate genetic counseling, and negligence in test tube conception have arisen in conjunction with the rapidly changing field of obstetrics and gynecology. Of equal importance has been a progressive increase in the number of medical liability cases alleging the improper use of or failure to employ certain diagnostic measures in the evaluation of pregnancy or specific gynecological conditions. Among the diagnostic measures that have become potent sources of potential malpractice problems is an old reliable ally—radiology.

201

The medical profession and the public at large have become increasingly aware of the potential hazards of diagnostic radiation, especially to the developing fetus. Accordingly, the general thrust in obstetrics has been to reduce the exposure of pregnant females to ionizing radiation. Professional medical organizations such as the American College of Obstetrics and Gynecology (ACOG) and the American College of Radiology (ACR) have established standards designed to protect the fetus while simultaneously providing for optimal use of diagnostic radiologic procedures.[1] Similarly, government agencies such as the National Council on Radiation Protection and Measurements (NCRPM) have set exposure limits for pregnant women and have established ideal time periods for radiographic examination of all women of childbearing age.[2] Addressing this latter concern, the NCRPM and the International Commission on Radiation Protection both advanced the notion that the risk of radiation injury to the fetus in utero could be minimized if women of childbearing age would undergo nonessential abdominal and pelvic radiologic examinations only during the first ten to fourteen days of the menstrual cycle and if they would avoid such examinations entirely during known pregnancy.[3] However, the validity of this approach has been seriously questioned. In fact, the ACOG-ACR policy statement on the subject refuted this recommendation and instead advocated:

1. individualization of radiologic examination;
2. proper utilization of the radiologist as a consultant, including assistance in evaluating x-ray exposure to the patient; and
3. better education of the patient about radiation risks in pregnancy.

In many jurisdictions, these recommendations would be admitted into evidence as the standard of care that should be adhered to by obstetrician-gynecologists and others who care for women in the childbearing years. Since the court might consider each of these a *duty* incumbent upon the physician, and failure to adhere to them a *breach* of that duty, I shall explore each recommendation, discussing not only the risks and recommendations involved in all such radiographic procedures, including nuclear medicine, but also the controversy surrounding those applications that some consider exotic or unnecessary.

Individualizing the Treatment

The possibility of future conception must be considered in the treatment of every patient with childbearing ability. Since obstetrician-gynecologists frequently act as primary care physicians for nonpregnant women of childbearing age, the responsibility falls on these practitioners to make sure their patients are only exposed to abdominal and pelvic x-rays when significant diagnostic information is likely to be obtained.

The admonition to recommend or request certain x-ray studies in women of childbearing age only with proper indication is implicit in the ACOG-ACR guidelines and suggests that physicians abandon the defensive practice of obtaining extensive radiographic studies on young and middle-aged women with minor gastrointestinal or pelvic complaints. Of particular concern is the indefensible practice of obtaining routine upper gastrointestinal, barium enema, and intravenous pyelogram studies on all patients who present with abdominal pain. Indeed, true defensive medical practice requires strict adherence to the establishment of the proper nexus between indication and radiographic procedure. Should the physician fail to heed this recommendation and continue to request unnecessary abdominal or pelvic x-ray studies, he may find his action identified as the *cause in fact* of the subsequent development of a childhood cancer in an offspring who was conceived or who was developing during the x-ray procedure. Conversely, of course, if an abdominal or pelvic radiographic study is indicated by history or physical findings, it should not be omitted because of fear of radiation exposure to a woman of childbearing ability, although nonradiation alternatives should be considered.

One prenatal radiographic procedure, x-ray pelvimetry, has been repeatedly challenged as an outmoded examination of dubious value. This argument represents a classic confrontation between risk and benefit. The risk, of course, is the radiation exposure to the intrauterine fetus, which can range from 1.1 to 4 rads depending on the number of repeat films required. As significant as this amount of exposure is, the real controversy relates to whether any significant benefit is derived from this procedure. At issue is whether the information obtained from pelvimetry is likely to alter the subsequent management of labor and delivery.

Varner et al. in a retrospective study conclude that information gained by pelvimetry is not usable in the prospective management of labor where there is a vertex presentation.[4] They do suggest that the procedure might be useful in prospective management of breech presentations. Their investigations indicate that ultrasound or abdominal scout film exams give esentially the same useful clinical information as pelvimetry. Pritchard and MacDonald state that the justification of x-ray pelvimetry will depend upon whether the decision to perform a cesarean section will be affected by the roentgen findings.[5] Since the morbidity associated with cesarean sections has markedly diminished, there is no longer a need to obtain pelvimetry as a defensive measure to justify this surgical procedure. They also point out that the probability of pelvic contractions or potential dystocia are adequate indications for pelvimetry.

There remain some radiologists who feel that modern radiation reducing equipment and techniques can significantly reduce the fetal radiation dose so that pelvimetry can be performed with relative safety.[6] The majority of clinicians, however, seem to agree with Laube et al., who concluded that pelvimetry was an unreliable tool in the diagnosis of cephalopelvic disproportion and, in general, had little usefulness in the management of labor.[7] Although no unified opinion exists concerning the indication for or the value of pelvimetry, most practitioners seem to agree that routine pelvimetry has no place in the modern practice of obstetrics. Clearly, in this circumstance, the risk outweighs the benefit. The development of leukemia in a child who had received intrauterine radiation from a pelvimetry procedure that was not indicated would certainly give rise to a question of the obstetrician's liability. Whether pelvimetry should be performed at all is a decision that must only be based on well-defined indications.

The more exotic radiographic procedures such as abdominal computerized axial tomography (CAT scan) should be avoided during the prenatal period unless the risk-benefit ratio clearly favors their employment. CAT scan procedures concentrate a large radiation exposure dose in a relatively small volume of tissue; thus, the fetus could conceivably receive an extremely high exposure dose during a maternal abdominal CAT scan. Deleterious results from nuclear magnetic resonance imaging have not been observed, but the relative infancy of this technology should dictate the same caution as that observed in CAT scanning.

Diagnostic radiation studies that do not involve the abdomen or the pelvis, e.g., chest x-rays, skull series, films of the extremities, do not usually need to be omitted during pregnancy since the beams can be circumscribed by collimation to the affected area or can be restricted from penetrating to the fetus by appropriate shielding. Nevertheless, even these x-ray studies should not be performed without proper indication to avoid the possibility of unnecessary scatter irradiation to the fetus.

The rapidly growing field of nuclear medicine offers another challenge to obstetrician-gynecologists who must be cognizant of the possible hazards of administering radioisotopes to pregnant women as well as to all women of childbearing age who could conceive in the future. Most of the concern with external irradiation is with the quantity of x-rays delivered to the fetus. Radioisotopes, on the other hand, present additional hazards related to the target organ for the specific isotope employed. For example, the fetal thyroid is at risk when therapeutic dosages of I-131 are administered to pregnant women. Damage including total destruction of the fetal thyroid have been reported from such therapy.[8] Even the use of diagnostic radioiodine in the form of I-125 or I-123 should be avoided during pregnancy since the possibility of carcinogenesis secondary to concentration of the radioisotope in the fetal thyroid cannot be excluded.

In evaluating the possible deleterious effects of radioisotopes, the physician must pay special attention not only to the form of the isotope and the target organ but also to the particle or type of radiation emitted and the half-life of the substance. In addition, the physician administering an isotope must be aware of whether the particular form crosses the placental barrier. The standard of care demands that the physician utilizing a particular nuclear medicine procedure have a thorough knowledge of all these variables, that the patient be informed about the potential risk to the fetus and the availability of alternative procedures, and that the patient give her informed consent. Accurate record keeping is a necessity since it might become necessary to verify to a court that this standard was met.

Consulting the Radiologist

The ACOG-ACR recommendation that the obstetrician-gynecologist obtain a preexamination consultation with the radiologist concerning proposed x-ray exposure to the patient may effectively preclude the obstetrician from asserting the defense that he was unaware of the significance of the exposure associated with a specific examination. The radiologist can help determine the dose that would be absorbed by the fetus if the pregnant woman were to be exposed to irradiation. The approximate fetal doses secondary to certain radiographic studies are listed in Table 1.[2]

The considerable variability in the actual fetal dose associated with a specific procedure is due to a number of factors, including the number of films used during a study and possible fluoroscopy exposure. Knowledge of these variables is essential so that the physician can properly counsel the patient concerning fetal irradiation absorption and possible

Table 1

Approximate Fetal Doses Secondary to Certain Radiographic Procedures

Procedure	Approximate Fetal Dose (Rads)	Additional Dose from Fluoroscopy
Lumbo-Sacral Spine Series	.275– .725	
Intravenous Pyelogram	.400– .600	
Upper Gastrointestinal Series	.175– .560	1.62
Barium Enema Examination	.800–1.000	2.16
Pelvimetry	1.1 –4.0	

complications. Consultation with a radiologist or radiation health physicist is necessary to obtain an accurate assessment of the fetal dose.

With the advent of new imaging techniques and the greater availability of exposure reducing equipment and examination methods, it is essential for the radiologist to become an active participant in decisions involving the obstetrical patient's exposure to radiation. The radiologist can select new rare earth screens, graphite cassettes, and high speed film to accomplish needed radiographic studies with a reduced fetal radiation dose.[6] Even if pelvimetry is required, the radiologist can overcome the problem of high fetal exposure dose through the use of CAT digital pelvimetry, which has a fetal absorbed dose only five percent of the dose generated by conventional x-ray pelvimetry.[9] Using information obtained from the patient's history and the referring physician's consultation, the radiologist can recommend and perform the proper procedure for the indication with the least amount of radiation exposure to both the pregnant woman and the fetus. Such a joint management approach will probably become the standard of care in the management of radiologic procedures involving the obstetrical patient.

Educating the Patient

Patient education must start prior to pregnancy since there is evidence that preconception maternal exposure to radiation may be associated with subsequent carcinogenesis in the offspring.[10] Further research is necessary to evaluate the validity of this observation and to gauge its impact on the standard of care which should be followed by the physician with regard to the disclosure of risk to females of childbearing age.

Once the patient has had her pregnancy confirmed, the obstetrician usually assumes responsibility for her prenatal care. Patient education must continue since multiple reports attest to the fact that irradiation of the intrauterine fetus increases the risk of development of leukemia and other types of cancer later in childhood.[11] Furthermore, the mutagenic properties of x-rays must be considered since prenatal irradiation has been associated with Down's syndrome and implicated in the production of certain congenital anomalies.[12] Should a child develop leukemia or be found to have a congenital defect, the parents will readily recall the mother's exposure to radiation during the pregnancy. Thus, the obstetrician providing prenatal care must meticulously observe the ACOG-ACR guidelines.

Once it has been determined that a woman has been exposed to irradiation while pregnant, an estimation must be made of the dose absorbed by the fetus and whether the dose was of such a magnitude as to warrant the recommendation of therapeutic abortion. The physician must counsel the patient on the advisability of seriously considering therapeutic abortion when the fetal dose is above the level generally accepted as possibly carcinogenic, teratogenic, or growth retardant. However, it is equally important for the physician to emphasize that the risk is extremely minimal when the calculated dose received by the fetus is well below this action level. Unnecessary or ill-advised therapeutic abortion could certainly engender legal action because of negligent counseling.

Although there is still considerable controversy about whether there is a threshold below which irradiation does not affect the fetus, most investigators concur that neither teratogenesis nor growth retardation is a significant risk after fetal irradiation absorption of less than 10 rads.[13] If this hypothesis is accepted and if the fetus has absorbed less than 10 rads, there would seem to be no justification for recommending therapeutic abortion based on a fear of teratogenesis or growth retardation. On the other hand, if it is determined that the fetus has absorbed more than 10 rads, the woman must be advised of the increased possibility of fetal growth retardation or fetal malformation; and although the physician is not obligated to recommend this course of action, therapeutic abortion should at least be discussed as an option. However, in either case, the patient must be provided with sufficient information to enable her to make an intelligent decision regarding the preservation or termination of her pregnancy.

The dose-dependent relationship between diagnostic radiation and subsequent teratogenesis or growth retardation is not noted with respect to carcinogenesis. The work of Stewart et al. suggests that a fetal dose as low as 1–2 rads increases the probability of the subsequent development of leukemia during childhood.[14] Also, unlike teratogenesis, which is stimulated by radiation during the early organogenic stage of pregnancy, leukemia and other childhood cancers are more prevalent following uterine irradiation late in pregnancy. Thus, carcinogenesis tends to be associated with procedures such as pelvimetry. In educating the pregnant woman about the risks inherent in these procedures, the clinician should refrain from issuing any assurance or guarantee to the pregnant woman that neoplasia later in childhood is unlikely because of the level of radiation absorbed by the fetus. Neither should the clinician precipitously recommend termination of pregnancy due to fear of delayed onset of carcinogenesis secondary to fetal irradiation. Indeed, as Brent points out, a policy of counseling abortion to those who have received intrauterine doses sufficient to eventuate in an increased risk of leukemia would result in the needless death of an enormous number of nonleukemic embryos to prevent one fetus from developing leukemia at a later age.[13] The clinician's dilemma can only be obviated by meticulous avoidance of unnecessary radiation to the pregnant female.

Summary

The prime duty of the clinician is to ensure that no intraabdominal irradiation is administered to the pregnant patient or indeed to any woman of childbearing age without appropriate indication. Should the patient receive abdominopelvic irradiation either inadvertently or because of some medical indication, the clinician has a duty to inform the patient of the possible consequences of this diagnostic encroachment upon the fetus. Indeed, the risks should be discussed with the patient prior to implementing any planned diagnostic x-ray examination of the abdomen or pelvis. Advice about aborting the fetus should be judiciously given, paying particular attention to the distinction between the teratogenic, carcinogenic, and growth retardant effects of irradiation. Strict adherence to the ACOG-ACR guidelines will help diminish the number of lawsuits filed alleging negligence with regard to fetal irradiation and, moreover, will permit better defense in those legal actions that are brought.

Diagnostic Ultrasound

The application of diagnostic ultrasound to the practice of obstetrics and gynecology is probably the single most important technological development that has occurred in this specialty in the past half century. The pioneering work of Donald and the Glasgow group in the late 1950s and early 1960s demonstrated the utility of this new diagnostic modality, the simplicity of its technical procedures, and its apparent noninvasive characteristics.[15,16] The past twenty years have seen an exponential growth in the numbers of physicians using ultrasound along with refinements of technique and increased sophistication of equipment. This pattern of growth is expected to continue as training becomes widespread and ultrasound equipment becomes universally available.[17]

The explosive introduction of this new technology with its impact on the fetus, the pregnant woman, and the gynecologic patient requires an evaluation of the legal implications of diagnostic sonography. Although I shall mainly address the legal issues surrounding the use of ultrasound in obstetrics, the principles involved can be readily transposed to gynecology.

Duty and the Standard of Care

A legal consideration of primary significance to cases involving ultrasonography is whether there is a duty owed by the defendant-physician to the plaintiff-patient. One tenet of the standard of care is that the health care provider, as a general rule, owes his patient the duty of being "possessed of ordinary skill and [employing] ordinary care in the patient's treatment" (p. 155).[18] Specialists such as obstetricians are held to a somewhat higher standard since their skills are expected to reflect their advanced training and since the quality of care they provide is consequently presumed to exceed that of the general physician. In a malpractice action, the entire case might turn on whether the obstetrician should or should not have recommended or obtained ultrasonography for his patient. Of central concern then are the accepted indications for obtaining sonographic evaluation of the pregnant female.

The medical literature is replete with recommended indications. Some of the most common include cephalometric assessment of fetal maturity and growth rates, determination of fetal viability, diagnosis of multiple pregnancy, congenital anomalies and incidental complications (e.g., fibroid, ovarian cysts), localization of the placenta, and determination of appropriate means of elective interruption.[19] The obstetrician who notes one of these indications and elects to procure a sonogram has fulfilled the duty required by the standard of care. However, if the obstetrician does not obtain a sonogram despite the presence of an acceptable indication, and if either the mother or the fetus sustain some injury, the issue of duty will assume paramount status. One clear example relates to those pregnancies in which amniocentesis is indicated. A court would probably find that an obstetrician has a duty to obtain sonographic placental localization before performing amniocentesis because of the hazards of fetal or placental damage and fetomaternal transfusion in the Rh-negative patient.

Does the obstetrician have a duty to obtain routine sonography of all gravid patients at some time during their pregnancies, even if none of the usual indications exist? Specifically, should pregnancy alone be considered an indication for sonography? While many obstetricians have certainly adopted this view, many others argue against mass screening of gravid patients purportedly for the detection of findings such as fetal anomalies.[19,20] These dissenters base their position on poor risk-benefit and cost-benefit ratios as well as the lack of qualified personnel to perform these duties.

Since such a divergence of opinion currently exists within the expert obstetrical community, the medical answer to this question is that a physician does not have a duty to perform routine obstetrical ultrasonography in the absence of specific indications. On the other hand, the legal answer to the question of the physician's duty vis-à-vis ultrasonography will be based on the adequacy of the ultrasonographer's and ultrasound technologist's training and the impact of local versus national standards of care.

The issue of adequate training is especially important in a field as new as diagnostic ultrasound. Because of its multidisciplinary usage, its apparent safety, and the rapid proliferation of both machines and users, the training requirements for both physicians and technicians lack uniformity and exactitude. Any radiographic technologist can hold himself out as an ultrasound technician after only minimal formal training. Similarly, a physician after a two-week crash course can assume the mantle of ultrasonographer. Professional medical and technical societies (e.g., American Society of Ultrasound Technical Specialists, American Board of Radiology) are attempting to establish guidelines and regulations designed to standardize training requirements in this specialty. The American Registry of Diagnostic Medical Sonographers (RDMS) has developed a registration program for ultrasound technologists which has varying requirements for general ultrasound course work dependent on the prior training of the technologist. Similarly the American Board of Radiology (ABR) promulgates a general training program leading to board certification in ultrasonography for physicians. However, state regulations of medicine and its ancillary disciplines vary significantly and impair these attempts at training uniformity. Nevertheless, standards of training that are considered necessary for competency will be advanced to the court by the expert witnesses for both the plaintiff and the defense; against these standards, the defendant physician's or technician's training will be measured.

A related issue that could arise in a malpractice action is the failure of the ultrasonographer to keep abreast of new developments. In the era of the bistable apparatus, the focus was on calculation of fetal age, evaluation of placental anomalies, and determination of fetal position. Recently, however, the development of gray-scale and real-time imaging has allowed the accurate evaluation of anomalous fetal growth, function, and development. Fetal anomalies can now be diagnosed at increasingly earlier stages of development, thus providing a more rational, informed basis for considering and/or recommending termination of the pregnancy. Whether a sonographer either used equipment that was inadequate by current standards or failed to maintain proficiency in performing or interpreting sonography could be significant issues in a malpractice action. Corollary issues include proper utilization of sources of knowledge and appropriate use of consultants, both of which will be considered in determining whether the practitioner met the standard of care.

Traditionally, the standard of care expected of a physician was determined by the locality rule. This rule stated that the degree of skill and learning possessed by a physician licensed in a state was measured against that of other reasonably prudent physicians in good standing in the community (or similar community); in addition, the physician was expected to apply that skill and learning, with ordinary and reasonable care, to those patients who came to him for treatment.[21] However, because of the standardization of ultrasound knowledge and the similarity in the skills of physicians and technicians who are engaged in this discipline in different parts of the country, the trend in most courts is to look to a minimal national standard for such specialists.[22] The standards advanced by the RDMS and the ABR are national in scope. Even in Kansas, a state that followed the locality rule, the state supreme court indicated that testimony about national standards was admissible as evidence in certain specific medical areas.[23]

Injury and Informed Consent

The prime issue driving a malpractice action is the injury that the plaintiff sustains as the result of the negligent action of the defendant, the so-called damages issue. But what are the possible damages that might arise in the obstetrical sonography setting? Certainly it has been amply demonstrated and is the belief of most physicians who work with it that utlrasound has no deleterious effects upon either the mother or the fetus. Nevertheless, certain disquieting research observations should inject a sense of caution before ultrasound is declared innocuous.

Mcintosh and Davey noted chromosome damage after exposure of cells in vitro to continuous-wave ultrasound of diagnostic intensities.[24] Although these findings have not been duplicated by other researchers, further studies are obviously necessary before concluding that diagnostic ultrasonography has no genetic effects.[25,26]

A committee of distinguished researchers in ultrasound who met at the Bureau of Radiological Health and exchanged information on the biological effects of ultrasound concluded that knowledge of the basic mechanisms of interaction of ultrasound with tissues is insufficient.[27] They were particularly concerned with the need for more epidemiological studies. At this meeting, William D. O'Brian, Jr., of the University of Illinois, reported an increase in clotting times in some experimental animals when insonated at reasonably low levels. O'Brian pointed out the seriousness of this threat to pregnant women in whom the blood is already in a natural state of hyperclottability. Other researchers at this meeting noted an inexplicable weight reduction in fetuses of experimental animals insonated at diagnostic levels. Basic questions of the mechanical effects of pulsed sound waves on human cells, including possible cavitation changes secondary to heating, remain unanswered. Recent articles indicate that the peak intensities at which diagnostic ultrasound is operated are considerably below the threshold for transient cellular cavitation.[28] Another group of researchers have an ongoing study to evaluate the possibility of weight reduction in children previously insonified in utero.[29] So far, the study has not substantiated any such weight reduction.

The assumption that ultrasound as a diagnostic tool is an inherently safe procedure should be made guardedly. No one can forget that x-rays were used for years before the dangers of irradiation to fetal or adult tissues were suspected. Diethylstilbesterol and thalidomide exposed the dangers of long- or short-term drug teratogenicity. Many of the genetic effects as well as some possible somatic effects might not become apparent until years after the ultrasound application. Consequently, a lawsuit might not be instituted until years after the ultrasound exposure when the injury and damage would be discovered. In view of the relatively short time obstetrical ultrasonography has been employed, the "jury is still out" about the effects of this physical modality on the fetus.

Since there is no certainty that ultrasonography is one hundred percent safe, it may be advisable to obtain the patient's informed consent prior to performing ultrasonic procedures. Under the doctrine of informed consent, the plaintiff-patient is required to establish:

1. the existence of a material risk that was unknown to the patient;
2. the failure of the physician to disclose it;
3. the fact that the patient would have chosen a different course if the risk had been disclosed; and
4. a resulting injury.[30]

Certainly this burden on the plaintiff is eased by the current practice of assuring the patient that ultrasound is completely safe. Should something untoward occur that could relate back to the sonographic procedure, the ultrasonographer might find himself accused of malpractice with the prime issue being lack of informed consent.

Respondeat Superior

A final issue that must be addressed in any discussion of the legal implications of ultrasonography relates to the legal concept of respondeat superior, i.e., any act of negligence attributed to an employee is imputed to his employer. In most cases, the actual sonographic procedure is performed by an ultrasound technician who is employed by a physician, a professional medical corporation, a clinic, or a hospital. Thus, if because of a technical error, a placenta previa is missed at ultrasonography and the resultant injury to fetus or mother engenders a malpractice action, the employing person or entity will be sued rather than or in addition to the technician. Moreover, under the borrowed servant doctrine, liability can extend even further. For example, the physician may be held accountable for the actions of the technician even if that person is an employee of the hospital. In addition, the physician's partner who does not participate in the alleged negligent act can nevertheless be sued because of the business relationship. Finally, even if the patient is referred to another specialist who actually provides the sonographic consultation and interpretation, the referring obstetrician may still be liable for any negligence that occurs, since it can be alleged that he knew or should have known of the ultrasonographer's incompetence.

Summary

My primary goal in raising some of the legal issues that are involved in this rapidly developing field is to sound a note of caution and prudence. Although I know of no recorded cases to date in either state or federal jurisdictions specifically alleging damage resulting from obstetrical sonography, little comfort can be taken from this fact since the same was also true of x-rays and many drugs at similar stages in their development. Therefore, I think that all who work in this field must observe certain precautions in order to reduce the possibility of future malpractice actions.

1. Obstetrical ultrasonography should be limited to specific indications accepted by a reasonable number of those in the field. Most ultrasonographers would agree that determination of fetal age, evaluation of intrauterine growth retardation, localization of placenta previa, and detection of congenital malformations are the chief indications for ultrasonography.
2. If one of these indications is present, ultrasonography should be employed in the diagnosis.
3. Routine obstetrical sonography should not be performed unless a definitive protocol has been established or it is part of an experimental program.
4. Ultrasonography should only be performed by adequately trained technologists and interpreted by properly trained ultrasonographers. Adequacy of training should be determined objectively, using standards set by professional and technical societies and/or by appropriate state regulatory agencies. ACOG recommends that a physician receive formal training in ultrasound at a medical center under the guidance of experienced professionals. They advocate training in ultrasonography be included in residency programs for obstetrics and gynecology as well as radiology. ACOG also supports accredited training programs and certifying examinations in ultrasonography for ultrasound technologists.[31]
5. The ultrasonographer must be aware of and adhere to the general standard of care in the community with regard to obstetrical

sonography. In addition, he must ascertain that this standard does not significantly deviate from the generally accepted national standard of the profession.

6. Continuing technical and professional education permits the technologist and physician to keep abreast of developments in the field of obstetrical ultrasonography. Special note must be made of research developments related to possible genetic or somatic damage resulting from diagnostic obstetrical ultrasound.

7. Even though no definite injurious complications of obstetrical sonography have been demonstrated yet, prudence suggests that the ultrasonographer consider obtaining the patient's informed consent before ultrasonography is performed. The patient should be told that no evidence of deleterious effects have been demonstrated so far, but, nevertheless, the procedure is limited to definitive indications and, in the patient's case, the benefit outweighs the known possible risks.

8. All those who employ ultrasound technicians (e.g., physicians, hospitals, clinics, professional corporations) must ascertain that these individuals have adequate training, credentials, integrity, and reliability since the employer will be held responsible for any negligence attributed to the technologist. Similarly, the referring physician should be certain of the qualifications of the ultrasonographer before referring patients to him. The guidelines proposed by such organizations as ACOG, RDMS, ABR, the Society of Diagnostic Medical Sonographers (SDMS), and the American Society of Ultrasound Technical Specialists (ASUTS) will be useful in this endeavor.

Obstetrical ultrasonography is an exciting and challenging addition to the tools used by the obstetrician in the management of pregnancy. As with all medical modalities, knowledge of the legal implications associated with this specialized technique is imperative for anyone who participates in obstetrical ultrasonography.

References

1. American College of Obstetricians and Gynecologists and American College of Radiology. Guidelines for diagnostic x-ray examination of fertile women. Washington, DC: American College of Obstetricians and Gynecologists, 1977.
2. National Council on Radiation Protection and Measurements. Medical radiation exposure of pregnant and potentially pregnant women (NCRP report no. 54). Bethesda, MD: Author, 1977.

3. International Commission on Radiation Protection. Protection of the patient in x-ray diagnosis (ICRP publication 16). New York: Pergamon Press, 1970.

4. Varner, MW, Cruikshank, DP, and Laube, DW. X-ray pelvimetry in clinical obstetrics. Obstet Gynecol 56(3):296, 1980.

5. Pritchard, JA and MacDonald, PC. Williams obstetrics, ed 16. New York: Appleton-Century-Crofts, 1980.

6. Bean, WJ and Rodan, BA. Pelvimetry revisited. Semin Roentgenology 17(3): 164, 1982.

7. Laube, DW, Varner, MW, and Cruikshank, DP. A prospective evaluation of x-ray pelvimetry. JAMA 246:2187, 1981.

8. Witkofsky, RL and Pizzarello, DJ. Basic radiation biology, ed 2. Philadelphia: Lea and Febiger, 1975.

9. Federle, MP. Pelvimetry, ultrasonography in obstetrics and gynecology. Philadelphia: WB Saunders, 1983.

10. Shiono, PH, Chung, CS, and Myrianthopoulos, NC. Preconception radiation, intrauterine diagnostic radiation and childhood neoplasia. JNCI 65(4):681, 1980.

11. Stewart, A and Kneale, GW. Radiation dose effects in relation to obstetric x-rays and childhood cancer. Lancet 1:1185, 1970.

12. Simpson, JL. Antenatal diagnosis of cytogenetic abnormalities. Clin Obstet Gynecol 24(4):1023, 1981.

13. Brent, RL. Irradiation in pregnancy. *In* Davis's gynecology and obstetrics, vol 2, rev ed, pp 26–27, 1976.

14. Stewart, A. Malignant diseases in childhood and diagnostic irradiation in utero. Lancet 2:447, 1956.

15. Donald, I. Investigation of abdominal masses by pulsed ultrasound. Lancet 1: 1188, 1958.

16. Donald, I. On launching a new diagnostic science. Am J Obstet Gynecol 103: 609, 1969.

17. Popp, L and Thomsen, R. Ultrasound in obstetrics and gynecology. New York: McGraw-Hill, 1978.

18. Meaney, T, Lalli, A, and Alfidi, R. Complications and legal implications of radiologic special procedures. St Louis: CV Mosby, 1973.

19. Scheer, K. Sonography as a routine obstetrical procedure. J Clin Ultrasound 5(2):101, 1977.

20. Sabbagha, R. Ultrasound in high risk obstetrics. Philadelphia: Lea and Febiger, 1979.

21. *Boyce v. Brown,* 51 Ariz 416, 77 P2d 455, 1938.

22. *Murphy v. Little,* 112 Ga App 517, 145 SE2d 760, 1965.

23. *Chandler v. Neosho General Hospital,* 223 Ks 1, 1977.

24. Mcintosh, IJ and Davey, DA. Chromosome aberrations induced by an ultrasonic fetal pulse detector. Br Med J 4:92, 1970.

25. Boyde, E. Chromosome breakage and ultrasound. Br Med J 2:501, 1971.

26. Brobaw, M, Blackwell, N, and Uhren, A. Absence of any observed effect of ultrasonic irradiation of human chromosomes. Br J Obstet Gynecol British Commonwealth 78:730, 1971.

27. Huerta, LK. Ultrasound—a completely safe method? App Radiology/Ultrasound, p 135, July–August 1971.

28. Carstensen, EC and Gates, AH. The effects of pulsed ultrasound on the fetus. J Ultrasound Med 3:145, 1984.
29. Lyons, EA, Coggrave, M, and Brown, RE. Follow-up study in children exposed to ultrasound in utero—analysis of height and weight in first six years of life. Presented at twenty-fifth annual meeting of AIUM, New Orleans, September 15–19, 1980.
30. *Miller v. Kennedy,* 11 Wash App, 272 P2d 852, affirmed 85 Wash 2d 151, 530 P2d 334, 1975.
31. American College of Obstetricians and Gynecologists. Diagnostic ultrasound in obstetrics and gynecology (ACOG technical bulletin 63). Washington, DC: Author, 1981.

Chapter 19

Medical-Legal Aspects of New Techniques to Create a Family[*]

George J. Annas and Sherman Elias

The acronyms IVF and ET conjure up a variety of images, from test tube babies to Steven Spielberg's Extraterrestrial. Indeed, it is sometimes difficult to separate science fiction from scientific reality. Nonetheless, the extracorporeal fertilization of a human egg followed by transfer to a human uterus and birth of a child has occurred in a number of countries around the world.[1] In vitro fertilization (IVF) and embryo transfer (ET) are now reality.[†] Most of us applaud this new technology along with the infertile couples who are able, with the help of IVF, to have their own offspring. But we also have some second thoughts. What are the broader implications of IVF? Do its benefits to individual couples outweigh its potential dangers to society? Should IVF be regulated?

---

[*] An earlier version appeared in Family Law Quarterly 17(2):199, 1983.

[†] *In vitro fertilization* is the extracorporeal fertilization of an ovum by sperm. *Embryo transfer* is the transfer of the fertilized ovum into the uterine cavity. An *ovum* is the female germ cell, egg cell, or gamete. An *oocyte* is an immature ovum. A *zygote* results from the union of a male gamete (sperm) and a female gamete (ovum), until it divides. An *embryo* is the product of conception from the moment of fertilization until about the end of the eighth week after fertilization. A *conceptus* is the sum derivatives of a fertilized ovum at any stage of development from fertilization until birth, including the extraembryonic membranes.

And if so, who should be the regulator and on what principles should legal rules be founded?

A 1979 study by the DHEW's Ethics Advisory Board (EAB Report) concluded that "development of a uniform or model law to clarify the legal status of children born as a result of *in vitro* fertilization and embryo transfer was desirable" (p. 113).[2]* Official agencies in Great Britain and Australia have already developed general guidelines for IVF research.[4-6] Scientist Clifford Grobstein and Congressman Albert Gore have suggested that the United States establish a Presidential Commission to review and monitor the development of IVF and make recommendations for appropriate legislation and regulation.[7,8] In his speech at the 1982 annual American Bar Association convention, Father Robert Drinan called the new reproductive technologies the greatest challenge facing the Family Law Section in the next twenty-five years.[9]

Modifications in reproductive methods have long been viewed as science fiction and have occasioned both fear and amazement. We are reminded of Orwell's *1984* in which artificial insemination by donor (AID) was mandatory, and sexual pleasure and the family were destroyed to help maintain the tension necessary in a society dedicated to perpetual warfare.[10] In Aldous Huxley's *Brave New World,* the family was also destroyed; but he portrayed a society controlled not by fear but by gratification and reinforcement.[11,12] Abolition of the family was followed by complete sexual freedom; but reproduction was handled by the state, in state hatcheries in which embryos were produced and monitored in an artificial environment:

> Of course, they didn't content themselves with merely hatching out embryos: any cow could do that. 'We also predestine and condition. We decant our babies as socialized human beings, as Alphas or Epsilons, as future sewage workers or . . .' He was going to say 'future world controllers,' but correcting himself, said 'future Directors of Hatcheries,' instead [p. 8].†

In both futuristic scenarios, the critical elements of governmental success were the separation of sex from reproduction and the abolition of the family. We will, of course, write our own future by our own actions, and IVF may not prove terribly crucial. Isaac Asimov, for example,

---

* A similar recommendation has been made by Noel P. Keane in regard to surrogate mothers.[3]

† Cf. *Lex Sexualis*: "A Number may obtain a license to use any other Number as a sexual product" (p. 22).[13]

doubts IVF will have much of an impact on society, and sees mainly advantages in complete ectogenesis:

> While test-tube fertilization may exist as an added option, it would not be surprising if it proved only minimally popular. We might, of course, go all the way and dispense with the human womb altogether . . . . The developing embryos would be under close observation at all times. Minor faults might be corrected. Embryos with serious deficiencies might be discarded. Some women might prefer the certainty of having healthy babies [p. 352].[14]

Whether one is of the catastrophy school or is a rose-colored-glasses optimist, we cannot permit major technological changes in the way families can be created to occur without careful thought. In this chapter, we shall provide an historical overview and a current state of the art regarding IVF and ET technology, review the legal issues these technologies raise, and consider potential problems that will arise should we not content ourselves with limiting IVF to married couples who are infertile because of the wife's obstructed fallopian tubes.

Historical Aspects

The first reports of mammalian IVF appeared in the scientific literature over a century ago, and the first successful ETs in rabbits were reported in 1890.[15,16] Freshly ejaculated sperm were rarely capable of fertilizing mature ova either in vivo or in vitro. In the early 1950s, researchers discovered that mammalian spermatozoa undergo a change during their passage through the epididymides that affects their maturation and enables them to fertilize ova.[17,18] This sperm maturation process, called *capacitation,* results from complex and not well understood physiological, biochemical, and morphological alterations in the sperm as they proceed through the tubules.

By the late 1960s, experimentation with rabbits resulted in consistent IVF successes. Sperm were recovered from the uterus of a mated animal after capacitation.[19,20] The rabbit ova were fertilized in vitro and allowed to progress to the four-cell stage. Subsequent transfer to rabbit oviducts resulted in an eighty percent pregnancy rate, and twenty percent live births.[21]

Most of the early technical advances in humans were made in England by Edwards and Steptoe, including fertilization of oocytes (ova removed directly from the ovary) matured in vitro, in vitro development of embryos to the blastyocyst stage, and collection of oocytes by laparoscopy.[22–24] In 1976, they reported a tubal ectopic pregnancy resulting from IVF; and in 1978, they announced the birth of the world's first IVF baby.[25,26] Shortly thereafter, other groups around the world began achieving successes; and in December 1981, the first IVF birth in the United States was announced at Eastern Virginia Medical School in Norfolk.[27,28]*

Medical Aspects

The state of the art has as many variations in procedure as there are clinics involved in IVF. What follows is a summary of general trends.

The protocol for management of patients participating in IVF depends on whether oocytes are collected during a natural or stimulated menstrual cycle. In the natural cycle approach, patients are not treated with hormones or drugs, and usually only one follicle will develop each ovulatory cycle. The timing of laparoscopy for oocyte recovery is usually determined by daily measurement of estrogen levels in the urine or plasma, and ultrasonographic evaluation of ovarian follicular size commencing on day nine or ten of the cycle.[30,31]† Twice-daily assays for urine or plasma samples for luteinizing hormone (LH) to ascertain a sustained increase in excretion rate is used to aid in the prediction of approaching ovulation.[32,33] Laparoscopy for oocyte aspiration is performed about twenty-eight hours after the onset of the LH surge, and a final ultrasonographic examination is performed immediately prior to the procedure to verify that an intact follicle is still present.

The first three children born using IVF were conceived following oocyte retrieval in the natural menstrual cycle. The disadvantages of attempting IVF with natural ovulatory cycles include:

1. usually only one preovulatory follicle is available for aspiration of an oocyte;
2. protracted monitoring is required to detect the LH surge;
3. the surgical team and facilities must be available twenty-four hours a day, seven days a week;

---

* On February 17, 1983, the sixteenth baby from the Virginia Clinic was born. It was a front-page story in its hometown of Minneapolis.[29]

† Laparoscopy is the visualization of the contents of the abdominal cavity by means of an optical instrument. This procedure is usually preceded by insufflation of the abdominal cavity with either carbon dioxide or nitrous oxide gas. Without intervention, the ovum would be extruded into either the peritoneal cavity or taken up by any remaining portion of the distal fallopian tube; thereafter, it would resorb (i.e., dissolve and assimilate).

4. the overall pregnancy rate is lower than with stimulated cycles where multiple follicles are available for aspiration; and

5. the stress of the situation often results in menstrual and ovarian follicle abnormalities.

Accordingly, almost all IVF centers now use stimulated ovulatory cycles.

For those women undergoing stimulated ovulations, successful recovery of mature oocytes from unruptured follicles depends on correctly judging two moments: when maturation is reached, and when follicular rupture spontaneously occurs. Clomiphene citrate (150 mg/day) is given on the fifth to ninth days of the menstrual cycle.* The growth and development of follicles is assessed by daily ultrasonographic monitoring beginning four days after the initiation of clomiphene administration.† When the dominant ovarian follicle reaches about 18 mm in diameter, estrogen levels are measured twice daily. In the normal cycle, serum levels of estradiol peak at thirty-three to thirty-six hours prior to the LH peak. Ovulation occurs after the LH peak. A plateau or slight decrease in estradiol is a signal from the ovaries to the hypothalamus/pituitary that the follicle is ready for ovulation. A blood sample is then taken for rapid assay of the LH level, and 4,000 to 5,000 international units of human chorionic gonadotropins (hCG) are administered. The hCG mimics the LH surge and thereby results in ovulation of the primed follicle. If the blood LH level is basal, laparoscopy is carried out thirty-six hours after the hCG injection.‡

Laparoscopy for oocyte recovery is usually performed under general anesthesia.§ The follicular fluid is immediately examined under a dis-

---

* Clomiphene citrate is an orally active agent with a chemical structure similar to estrogen; however, clomiphene itself does not have significant steroid effects. The mechanism of action is to cause the hypothalamus to perceive the level of estrogen in the circulation to be low. This obscured perception of low estrogen leads the hypothalamus to signal the pituitary gland to stimulate the ovarian follicular apparatus. As in the normal cycle, the rise in follicle-stimulating hormone secreted from the pituitary stimulates a set of follicles to begin growth and maturation.

† If the follicles appear small (i.e., less than 14 mm), additional stimulation in the form of human menopausal gonadotropins is possible.

‡ If the preinjection LH level is raised, indicating that the woman's own LH surge is under way, the cycle is abandoned, since the timing of ovulation is uncertain. LH rises spontaneously in about ten percent of cases.[34]

§ The pneumoperitoneum (insufflation of the abdominal cavity) is created with a gas mixture of ninety percent nitrogen, five percent carbon dioxide, and five percent oxygen to avoid exposing the oocyte to 100 percent carbon dioxide which may be harmful because of the tendency to develop acidic follicular fluid.[30] This gas mixture must be used with great caution because of the potential danger of gas embo-

secting microscope, and where no oocyte is found, the follicle is rinsed with culture medium and the contents are reaspirated.* With stimulated cycles, several ovarian follicles are usually available for aspiration.

A semen specimen is obtained five to six hours following oocyte retrieval and allowed to liquify for about thirty minutes.† After the semen specimen is washed and incubated for two hours, 0.5 to 1 million spermatozoa are added to each oocyte for eighteen hours.‡ The oocytes are then transferred into growth medium and allowed to incubate for an additional twenty hours. About thirty-eight to forty hours after insemination, the fertilized ovum's development is assessed.

Pregnancies have been achieved following transfer of two-cell to sixteen-cell embryos, but the optimal stage for ET has not yet been determined.[38,39] Most investigators perform ET about forty-eight hours after laparoscopy.§ The Virginia researchers emphasize the importance of transferring more than one conceptus per cycle if possible. In their limited 1981 series, with the transfer of a single conceptus, the pregnancy rate was thirteen percent (two of fifteen cases); with two conceptuses, it was thirty-one percent (four of thirteen cases).‖

Following ET, the patient is usually required to remain at bedrest for about twenty-four hours. Blood samples are obtained commencing seven days after laparoscopy and assayed for plasma progesterone and

---

lism. Usually three abdominal punctures are required—one for the laparoscope, another for a probe to manipulate the ovary to gain access to all its surfaces, and a third for the aspirating instrument. A single-lumen Teflon-lined needle of about 1.5 to 2.0 mm in internal diameter employing a 100 mm mercury vacuum is utilized for follicle aspiration.[35]

* If the follicle has already ruptured at the time of laparoscopy, the follicle and the pouch of Douglas (area behind the uterus) are aspirated in an attempt to recover the oocyte. The follicular fluid and oocyte must be kept at a constant temperature of 37°C in a water bath.

† During this time the oocytes are allowed to incubate at 37°C in culture medium without spermatozoa which allows completion of the maturation of the oocytes.[36,37]

‡ If necessary, frozen semen may be used for insemination after washing.

§ The woman is premedicated with a sedative or hypnotic agent and placed in either the left-lateral position or the lithotomy position. After the cervix and the upper vagina are cleaned with tissue culture medium, a Teflon-lined catheter with a hole in the side of the tip is introduced through the cervical canal into the uterine cavity for ET. A column of air precedes the fluid containing the embryo. After the embryo is injected, a delay of about one minute before removal of the catheter is recommended to facilitate dispersal of the embryo. Finally, the catheter is inspected under a dissecting microscope to assure that the embryo has been expelled.

‖ On two occasions, they transferred three conceptuses, with one resulting pregnancy.[28]

hCG to monitor continued embryonic growth. Ultrasonographic studies are performed beginning about eight weeks gestation to determine the number of fetuses and to continue monitoring fetal viability and growth. Otherwise, management of the pregnancy is routine.

Results of IVF and ET Programs

Assessing the success rates of IVF and ET programs is difficult because of varying definitions of *success,* e.g., some investigators report an ectopic pregnancy as successful. The success rate is also likely to vary between programs and even within a single group because of the complex variables involved. Some investigators base their success rate on pregnancies per ET. Another method is pregnancies per laparoscopy.

A recent survey indicated that, in England, Steptoe and Edwards have performed about 600 laparoscopies for oocyte retrieval with a pregnancy rate of approximately sixteen percent.[40] In Melbourne, Australia, at the Royal Women's Hospital, about 300 laparoscopies were performed in 1981 with only seventeen pregnancies (five percent); only four continued beyond sixteen weeks gestation. At the Queen Victoria Hospital in Melbourne, the pregnancy rate ranged between ten percent and twenty percent, depending on the drugs used to stimulate the cycles (the number of laparoscopies was not quoted). At the University of Southern California, Los Angeles, twenty-five laparoscopies have been performed with four pregnancies.[34] At the Eastern Virginia Medical School, seven pregnancies were reported following ninety-six laparoscopies.[28]

Among the pregnancies established following IVF, there have been two abnormalities reported: a spontaneous abortion of a triploid fetus,* and the birth of a child with transposition of the major vessels of the heart.[41,42] The limited available data, thus, do not suggest an increased frequency of congenital abnormalities among IVF conceptuses. However, continued monitoring is mandatory to establish accurate frequencies. In experienced IVF clinics, the frequency of spontaneous abortions also does not seem to be in excess of that expected for natural conceptions in a population of infertility patients (twelve to eighteen percent).[43] Finally, the several tubal pregnancies reported following IVF are not unexpected, since most of these women have remnants of severely damaged fallopian tubes which might predispose toward ectopic implantations.[25,44]

---

* A triploid has sixty-nine chromosomes rather than the normal number of forty-six.

Legal Aspects

IVF has been the subject of a major federal report, more than a dozen law review articles and notes, and one civil lawsuit.[2,45-56]* There are some professional guidelines in specific countries and at specific medical institutions, but there have been no state or federal statutes or regulations adopted that are supportive of IVF.[4-6,40]† Even though the medical and technical aspects of IVF are still evolving, there is much more consensus regarding the technical aspects than its legal aspects. In the remainder of this chapter, we shall review the current legal status of IVF and make some suggestions regarding future regulation.

The Status of the Embryo

The most ethically and politically controversial aspect of IVF is the status of the embryo. Some opponents argue that a fertilized egg is a human being and that failure to reimplant it should be considered murder.[40,58] An analogous view has been put into an Illinois statute that requires the physician who performs IVF to assume the "care and custody" of the embryo and to be subject to the penalties of the child abuse statute should any harm befall it.‡ The constitutionality of the

---

 * In *Del Zio v. Presbyterian Hospital,* a jury returned a verdict for $50,000 in favor of prospective parents who sought recovery for their pain and suffering caused by the deliberate destruction of a potential embryo (the sperm had been introduced into the dish containing the oocyte, but fertilization had not yet been confirmed) by the hospital's chief of obstetrics and gynecology.[54] The chief contended that the IVF procedure represented risky experimentation that had not been approved by the hospital's IRB.

 † Illinois has a statute directly on IVF (Illinois Rev Stat chapter 38, section 81-26 [7]). Other states have fetal research statutes that might be interpreted to affect IVF. The Massachusetts fetal research statute, for example, is broad enough to encompass research with embryos (Massachusetts General Law chapter 112, section 12J) and prevented any IVF activity in Massachusetts until March 1983 when the district attorney for the district in which Boston's major teaching hospitals are located said that if all the fertilized eggs used were implanted in the woman, IVF "would appear to be in total compliance with the law" (p. 1).[57]

 ‡ "Any person who intentionally causes the fertilization of a human ovum by a human sperm outside the body of a living human female shall, with regard to the human being thereby produced, be deemed to have the care and custody of a child for the purposes of Section 4 of the Act to Prevent and Punish Wrongs to Children, approved May 17, 1977, as amended, [Illinois Rev Stat chapter 23, section 2354 (1981)] except that nothing in that Section shall be construed to attach any penalty to participation in the performance of a lawful pregnancy termination [Illinois Rev Stat chapter 38, section 81-26 (7)]."

statute has been unsuccessfully challenged by a physician and his patients, a married couple, who allege that it prevents them from employing IVF in violation of the couple's constitutional right to privacy and that it is unconstitutionally vague. The essence of the argument is that the statute's primary purpose is to prohibit IVF and that such a prohibition cannot be constitutionally accomplished by protecting embryonic life against the mother's interests prior to viability.[59] This argument seems correct. The United States Supreme Court has ruled that there is a right not to procreate, and this right seems best understood as a right not to have the state interfere in procreative decisions. The right at stake is privacy, and it seems that the decision by an infertile couple, made in concert with their physician, to undergo IVF for the purposes of having a child, should be constitutionally protected. The state has no obligation to foster IVF research or to pay for IVF procedures with Medicaid funds, but it does have an obligation not to interfere with such procedures unless it can demonstrate a compelling interest.[46,60–63]

The only candidate for a compelling interest seems to be preserving respect for human life by respecting the embryo. Replanting the embryo would accomplish this objective; but what about discarding *excess* embryos? The Illinois attorney general, Neil Hartigan, and the state's attorney of Cook County, Richard M. Daley, defended the statute by interpreting it in a way that would not interfere with the IVF procedure contemplated by the plaintiffs. They specifically limited physician custody to the preimplantation period and limited the duty imposed on the physician as refraining "from willfully endangering or injuring" the conceptus. Should the conceptus be found defective and its development terminated for this reason, the defendants interpreted this decision as a lawful termination of pregnancy on the part of the physician.* In his memorandum opinion, Judge Joel Flaum adopted the defendants' interpretation of the statute and dismissed the case for lack of subject matter jurisdiction, since under that interpretation there was nothing

---

* The defendants did not, however, explain why the same logic regarding pregnancy termination would not apply to an apparently normal conceptus. The opinions set forth in the defendants' memorandum detailing their interpretation of the statute do not have the force of law. Nevertheless, Judge Flaum noted in his decision, "there is a long history of their use in this State which suggests that they are far more than the personal reflections of the current office holder. Indeed, the opinions can have collateral effects for state officers who rely on or ignore them and the opinions are accorded considerable weight in the courts when a question of first impression is raised regarding the construction of an Illinois statute."[64]

to prohibit the plaintiffs from proceeding with IVF and, therefore, no case or controversy. As to the issue of multiple embryos, the judge decided it was not properly before him since the plaintiffs did not indicate they would use superovulation.[17,18]

All commentators have agreed that the embryo, even if not accorded human status, is worthy of respect. Two possible compromise solutions now exist. The first is to reimplant all embryos into the woman. This solution, which seems reasonable if only two or three are involved, now seems to have been adopted by many clinics since it seems to increase the probability of a pregnancy.[28] The second solution is more controversial. Excess embryos would be frozen.* This solution permits their use in future cycles, should the initial attempts fail, and in future pregnancies, but also raises the possibility of use in another couple or in a surrogate mother. We discuss the surrogate and donor scenarios later.†

Indications

Medically, IVF and ET have been developed primarily to permit married couples who are infertile, due to the wife's irreparable fallopian tube disease, to have children. IVF may also prove useful in cases where the husband has a low sperm count or other semen abnormalities, such as low sperm motility. A more controversial indication is idiopathic infertility, where evaluation of the couple (i.e., history, physical examination, laparoscopy, testing of fallopian tube patency, endocrine profiles, semen analysis, etc.) reveals no cause for infertility. An estimated ten to fifteen percent of infertile couples fall into this category. Possible explanations include immunologic factors, undiagnosed abnormalities of oocyte or sperm transport, undefined physical or chemical barriers preventing sperm penetration of the ovum, genetic abnormalities, and unrecognized uterine abnormalities. Virtually all cases of infertility, exclusive of intractable anovulation and those women without a uterus, are potential candidates for IVF.

Legally and ethically, who should be considered a candidate for IVF and ET? For example, should single women with fallopian tube disease be considered candidates for the procedure? This question should probably be answered the same as the question of whether single women

---

* This procedure is currently being used in Australia.

† A related issue to IVF is the use of *spare* embryos for research purposes.[65–67] Discussion of this aspect is beyond the scope of this chapter.

should be considered candidates for AID, i.e., whether medical technology should be used to aid in the creation of single-parent families.* The EAB Report recommended that IVF be restricted to married couples.[2] In Australia, the recommendation is even more restrictive: while acceptable to favor married couples who have had children during the experimentation phase, after IVF becomes established procedure, priority should be given to those married couples who have not had any children.[40] This issue needs to be resolved on a broader base than medical practice since the issues involved are not medical. Should we use technology to encourage single-parent families? To create children for lesbian couples? Transsexual couples?[69,70] The answer to these questions is not obvious, but the issues are complex enough that, at least until the medical aspects of IVF are standardized, it seems reasonable to put the burden of proof on those who do not want to restrict IVF to married couples and who contend that children do as well in alternate family settings as they do in traditional ones.

Selection of Patients

Couples seeking IVF must undergo genetic evaluation. For example, Jewish couples should be screened to determine their carrier status for Tay-Sachs disease. If both are carriers, antenatal diagnosis is appropriate. There are relatively few medical contraindications to IVF,† although there is a need for psychological counseling due to the high failure rates.[38] A screening laparoscopy should be performed to determine whether the ovaries are accessible for oocyte collection.‡ At least

---

* Apparently only about ten percent of practitioners of AID will use it for single women.[68] While there have been no decided lawsuits on this question, after the filing of a lawsuit brought on behalf of a thirty-six-year-old divorcee who applied for artificial insemination and was rejected because she was single, Wayne State University agreed in 1980 to include single women in its artificial insemination program.[3]

† Some investigators have reservations about using women over thirty-five because of the increased risk of chromosomal abnormalities, such as Down's syndrome.[41] However, pregnancies can be monitored via midtrimester amniocentesis. Because of theoretical risks, some investigators recommend that all couples undergoing IVF should be counseled about amniocentesis for prenatal diagnosis regardless of age. Although the number of pregnancies following IVF are still limited (under 200), the risk of abnormalities among infants born following IVF does not appear to be in excess of that expected for normal fertilization. For obstetrical reasons, women with serious medical illnesses (e.g., severe diabetes mellitus or heart disease) should be discouraged from attempting pregnancy.

‡ The screening laparoscopy may be timed at midcycle since there is a possibility that a mature ovarian follicle may be aspirated at this initial investigation. If only

at this stage of its development, there is probably no more right to be a recipient of IVF technology than there is a right to receive an artificial heart or a heart transplant.[71] If a medical facility does have a set of screening guidelines, however, it must apply them fairly and reasonably.

Informed Consent

IVF is still an experimental procedure, so all of the rules relating to consent to human experimentation should be observed.* The wife's consent must be both informed and knowledgeable. Since IVF involves the use of the husband's sperm, he should also be fully informed and give his own consent to the entire procedure. The would-be child, of course, cannot consent; therefore, the child, it has been suggested, might be able to sue the physician and/or its parents for wrongful life should it be born defective.[55,73,74] We do not believe any wrongful life lawsuit by or on behalf of the child should be permitted in the absence of negligence on the part of the physician or clinic.† Nonetheless, since

---

one ovary is accessible, IVF can be restricted to cycles when mature follicles are developing in that ovary, as determined by ultrasonographic monitoring. Occasionally, intraabdominal adhesions or disease (e.g., endometriosis) may necessitate a laparotomy to free one or both ovaries to permit future ovarian accessibility. This intervention usually involves suturing the supporting ovarian ligaments to the lateral pelvic wall to stabilize the ovary in the anterior portion of the pelvis.

* While there are no specific federal regulations applying to IVF, after implantation the regulations on fetal research apply, and prior to implantation the suggestions of the EAB Report should be followed.[2,45,72]

† The basic reason for not permitting suits against the parents is twofold: (1) the parents are obligated to care for the child in any event, and unless they give the child up for adoption, the money a child might obtain in such a suit would be used to care for the child anyway; (2) such a suit would be disruptive of family life. It has been argued that no lawsuit for wrongful life should lie against a negligent physician either, because the critical element of such a lawsuit is the contention that but for the negligence of the physician, the child would not have been born at all (e.g., if the physician had properly inspected the embryo or properly performed amniocentesis the physician would have recognized a significant defect and counseled the mother to abort). The argument is that it is impossible to assess damages since this requires a comparison of life with a defect versus no life at all. The contrary argument is that the child is not arguing that it would rather be dead, but is arguing that given a choice it would have chosen not to exist. Since it was not given that choice and does exist, it should be compensated for a wrong done that led to its defective existence. The counterargument is that it was not the wrong that led to its defect; it was defective to begin with and so never had the option of being born healthy, only of not being born or being born defective. Since the physician did not cause the defect, he should not have to pay for it. This seems correct in general; nevertheless, recent cases in

the would-be child is an innocent third party to the IVF agreement between the parents and the physician, we believe that all involved have an ethical obligation to protect the would-be child's interests.[77] As Hans Tiefel argues, "No one has the moral right to endanger a child while there is yet an option of whether the child shall come into existence" (p. 3238).[70] The state can also properly step in to regulate IVF on the basis of protecting the would-be child's interests in instances where there may be a conflict between the interests of the would-be child and those of the parents and physician. Tiefel continues, "We must weigh the chances for the well-being of the child while we yet have a choice about initiating this life. Would-be parents have moral obligations to a would-be child."

There is unlikely to be any conflict between the best interests of the child and a married couple applying for IVF, even using donor oocytes. However, should the embryo be transferred not to the wife, but to a surrogate childbearer (popularly referred to as a surrogate mother) who bears the child for the wife, many potential problems arise.

Donor Oocyte Embryos

Donor oocytes fertilized in vitro with the recipient's husband's sperm or by donor sperm may be used for embryo transfer in the following situations:

1. the recipient lacks ovaries either because of a genetic disorder (e.g., gonadal dysgenesis) or because they have been surgically removed;
2. the ovaries are inaccessible for oocyte retrieval due to pelvic disease; or
3. premature menopause.

Either the ovulatory cycle of the recipient must be synchronized with that of the donor by hormonal manipulation, or deep-frozen embryos could be thawed and transferred at the appropriate time.*

California and Washington have upheld wrongful life suits on the basis that special damages can be proven, and the physician was in fact negligent, and if damages were not awarded we would have a wrong without a remedy. The argument in favor of awarding damages is primarily an insurance argument and a deterrent argument (we want someone to help pay for the child's medical care, and we want to deter negligence on the part of physicians and clinics). Since the courts are split (and seem likely to remain so), legislative action may be appropriate.[75,76]

* Alan Trounson, working at Monash University, Melbourne, Australia, acknowl-

The issues raised by the use of donor oocytes are analogous to those raised by AID.* In each case, a human is donating or selling his or her gametes for the purpose of enabling a member of the opposite sex to have a child. The primary differences involve the risks to the woman in having the oocyte removed and the much smaller number of oocytes a woman can donate (usually only one at a time) as compared with the number of sperm a man can donate. These differences suggest that:

1. oocyte donors should be screened much more carefully than sperm donors have been, since they should not be put at any risk if their oocytes are unlikely to aid (and may even be harmful to) the donee;
2. oocyte vendors, if paid, should be paid substantially more for their oocytes than sperm vendors are paid for their sperm; and
3. complete medical records should be maintained on the donor or vendor so that she can be matched with resulting children should a genetic disease or disorder appear.

Also, it may be in the interest of the child to be told the identity of his or her genetic mother, and if this can be demonstrated, the information should be available.†

While donor oocytes have the advantage that they can be fertilized with the husband's sperm, they may be difficult to obtain. Accordingly, there may be some incentive to freeze excess embryos obtained from IVF procedures and offer them to infertile couples as a form of prenatal adoption.‡ This is the next step on the slippery slope of external fer-

---

edged that "eggs had been donated in 10 to 15 women who had no ovaries, who had ovaries from which eggs could not be obtained, or who had genetic diseases that could be passed on. He said that he preferred not to comment on the success of the transplants, but he did comment that 'this looks like a technique which will work'" (p. 5).[78]

* These issues as they relate to AID are discussed elsewhere.[79]

† Current evidence is insufficient to conclude that access should be mandatory, but while studies go on, the information should be retained.

‡ To increase the flexibility of the timing of ET, techniques for embryo preservation are required. Indeed, Trounson and Conti have suggested that in vitro clinics may have an obligation to develop preservation methods to be employed in circumstances where embryos cannot be transplanted—because of illness or unexpected difficulty— or where excess embryos develop but are not disposed of or used for other purposes.[43] Preliminary investigations into the deep-freezing (cryopreservation) of human embryos indicate that following thawing continued growth and development in culture is possible.[80] Trounson and Wood have reported the transfer of two such embryos in women without resulting pregnancies.[38] Although animal data have not indicated

tilization about which individuals such as Leon Kass and Paul Ramsey have expressed grave fears.[86–88] Why? The argument, on one level at least, is that there is a difference in kind, not degree, between oocytes, sperm, blood, and kidneys, on the one hand, and an embryo, on the other. There is general societal agreement that it is morally and legally wrong to sell a human being. The issue is whether sale or commercialization in embryos will lead to a general feeling that embryos, fetuses, and children are commodities and can be treated like commodities—e.g., defective children returned, differential fees charged for higher quality embryos. One can envision catalogs of embryos, with pictures and personal histories of the sperm and oocyte vendors, from which prospective parents can choose their own dream child.* Such a development does not strike us as an advance and certainly moves IVF outside the realm of medical intervention for specific disease conditions and into the realm of commercial products available for a wide variety of personal reasons. While not quantifiable, the dangers inherent in marketing embryos seem to us sufficiently grave to suggest a policy that prohibits traffic in them.†

---

an increased risk of fetal abnormalities as compared to nonfrozen embryos, extrapolation to human embryos may not necessarily be valid. Thus, a high degree of caution must be exercised prior to applying cryopreservation to human embryos. Craft and Yovich state that "90% of patients undergoing elective sterilization are prepared to donate ova for an approved research study and at least half of these would allow ova to be donated to an infertile couple" (p. 642).[81]

* It has been suggested that sperm banks market directly to women.[85]

† While beyond the scope of this chapter, it should be noted that IVF may also lead to the development of microsurgical techniques to manipulate defective embryos. It is now well established that among natural human fertilizations about fifty percent of first trimester spontaneous abortions are chromosomally abnormal.[86] Based upon the assumption that fifteen percent of pregnancies result in spontaneous abortions, one can conclude that about seven percent of all human conceptions are chromosomally abnormal. Presumably, a similar frequency of chromosomally abnormal embryos exists among those originating from IVF. Thus, if chromosomal studies could be performed on the embryo prior to transfer, one could avoid transferring a chromosomally abnormal conceptus which would be destined to either abort or result in a stillborn or liveborn child with a chromosomal abnormality. Using microsurgical techniques, one or several cells could be removed from the early embryo for chromosomal analysis. Because cells from such early embryos are thought to be totipotential, it would not be unreasonable to assume that continued normal development would ensue after such sampling. It has been demonstrated in animal studies that genetically identical offspring can result from the division of two-cell and four-cell embryos.[87] Similar microtechniques could be developed to detect other genetic disorders (e.g., inborn errors of metabolism).

Finally, cells could be incorporated into early embryos to complement for a genetic

234 CONFRONTING THE MALPRACTICE CRISIS

Surrogate Childbearers

These techniques offer potential parents the opportunity to have the embryo transferred to the uterus of a surrogate childbearer. While this option has not yet been exercised to our knowledge, it could be used for three medical indications and one personal one:

1. hysterectomy;
2. abnormal uterus (e.g., a bicornuate uterus);
3. Mullerian aplasia (i.e., congenitally absent uterus); and
4. a preference not to undergo the physical experience of pregnancy.

With the inclusion of the latter, IVF could potentially be available to all women who can produce oocytes. The question is whether it should be.

IVF itself closes a circle: oral contraceptives effectively separated sex from having children; IVF separates having children from sex. Surrogate childbearers go the next step: procreation is divorced not only from sex, but also from any anticipation of child rearing. The experience of surrogate childbearers in the United States to date (using AID, not IVF) strongly suggests that this method of procreation should be discouraged by medical and legal practitioners alike.

A recent chapter in the surrogate mother saga—where real life makes the soap operas appear pallid—involved Alexander Malahoff who contracted with Judy Stiver to be artificially inseminated with his sperm and bear him a child. Malahoff was separated from his wife and hoped the baby might help reunite them. The child was born January 10, 1983, with microcephaly. Mrs. Stiver immediately disavowed any responsibility, claiming the child was not hers. Malahoff likewise refused to take the child, claiming it was not his. Blood and tissue typing tests later upheld Malahoff. Prior to the insemination they had entered into a contract, the only instrument that in any way defined their respective rights and responsibilities, and one that legal scholars believe is probably unenforceable in a court. The contract specified that Stiver was to refrain from having intercourse with her husband for thirty days after the insemination, but remarkably mentioned nothing about the days

---

deficiency. For example, if the metabolic pathway of an embryo was known to lack a given enzyme, a cell (or cells) known to have that enzyme functioning properly could be transplanted into the embryo. Alternatively, pieces of DNA could be spliced into the genome of the embryo to correct for a particular genetic disorder. Such recombinant DNA research has already proved useful in bacterial systems to produce desired gene products such as insulin.[88,89]

prior to the insemination. While Malahoff's problem was resolved—he is quoted as saying, "Instead of a baby, I end up with a lawyer" (p. 76)[90]—ours is not as easily solved.[91] Roger Rosenblatt notes,

> A procedure has been devised in which a human being is literally conceived as a manufactured product. Therefore, consciously or not, all the participants in that procedure tend to regard the product either as the flower of a growth industry or, if a flap appears, as industrial waste [p. 90].[92]

Attorney Noel Keane, who considers himself the father of surrogate motherhood, describes in his recent book the individuals involved in the first surrogate cases he handled.[3]* In one of his first cases, the surrogate was an alcoholic lesbian who extorted money from the couple both before and after the birth of the child, who was born with fetal alcohol syndrome. In another, the couple in the market for a surrogate was infertile because the woman was a transsexual who had had a sex change operation. In that case, the surrogate decided to keep the child, and a court battle for joint custody began between the New York couple and the California surrogate.† A third involved a single man who wanted to have a son but did not want to get married.

Attorney Keane concludes from his experiences that state legislation is necessary to regulate the procedure.[3,96] Legislation has already been introduced in a number of states, including Michigan.‡ But before we rush to legislate, we should be clear on the issues at stake. A full

---

* Noel Keane has argued that single males are legally in a very good position to pay for the services of a surrogate, even in states that prohibit payment for adoptions because the father-sperm donor is the biological father of the child so no adoption is required on his part. Keane has also taken a client who wishes to donate his sperm to an "infertile white couple" who would then have "his" child and raise it themselves. He would set up a trust fund for the child ($20,000) and would "be like an uncle to it." Keane acted as the man's attorney and placed ads for him in the *Detroit Free Press* and *The Village Voice*. After choosing the couple, they decided not to enter into an elaborate written agreement because, according to Mr. Keane, "They met and came to trust each other" (p. 3).[93] While there is no law prohibiting such an arrangement, it does not strike us as one lawyers ought to be involved in or encourage since the effects on the child and the family are very problematic, and the motivations of the donor-uncle bizarre at best. Indeed, the uncle-sperm-donor case merely serves to underline the reproductive free-for-all attitude that seems to say any way to have a child is legitimate no matter how bizarre.

† In a hearing prior to the birth, the judge ruled that the surrogate could name the child, but that custody would not be determined until after the child was born. In a settlement agreement, the surrogate retained custody and the father was acknowledged on the birth certificate.[94,95]

‡ On February 8, 1983, Representative Richard Fitzpatrick of Battle Creek introduced HB 4114, a "Bill to Regulate Surrogate Parenting." His proposal, which seems

discussion of them is beyond the scope of this chapter, and many others have written about regulating surrogate motherhood.[3,101-106] We suggest, nonetheless, that two interrelated concerns should be paramount in any legislative or regulatory scheme: the best interests of the child, and minimizing the commercial aspects of the transaction.

To address the first issue, potential parents and society must view the would-be child not only as the end product of a surrogate transaction, but as the party who deserves the most protection because the child cannot speak for itself or represent its own interests, and because we have an obligation to the child to ensure that actions are not taken when there is good reason to believe they will be harmful to the child. The fact the would-be child does not exist when the contract is entered into and, therefore, cannot be said to possess any rights does not diminish our ethical obligation to take all reasonable steps to protect the would-be child's welfare.[77]* To give one example, current surrogate contracts do not generally take into account the child's possible desire to know the identity of its biological mother.[3,107] We suggest that the child should have a contractual right to this information, although the exercise of this right could be postponed until the child reached the age of majority. Likewise, the would-be child would probably prefer to have two parents who have accepted legal responsibility prior to birth and who would likely provide more financial and psychological protection than would a single parent.

The second issue has played the most prominent role in the surrogate debate to date—baby selling. The question involves the application of black-market baby statutes, which most states have, that forbid the payment of money to a woman who is placing her child for adoption. Kentucky law, for example, invalidates consent for adoption or the filing of a voluntary petition for termination of parental rights prior to the fifth day after the birth of a child and also prohibits remuneration related to adoption. Since the remuneration provision applies only to

---

drafted primarily to deal with cases like Malahoff, would clarify parental identity of the parties involved, and legalize the procedure. Senator Connie Binsfield of Maple City will reportedly introduce legislation to outlaw surrogate arrangements in Michigan.[97-99] "If the state of Michigan is ultimately going to recognize surrogate parent arrangements, comprehensive legislation is needed to resolve profound societal concerns related to the rights, obligations and interests of all parties."[100] Other states with pending legislation include South Carolina (HB 3491), which would regulate surrogate agreements, and Alabama (HB 593), which would outlaw them.

* "It makes good moral sense never to beget offspring when would-be parents cannot reasonably ensure a future child a fair chance at health" (p. 3238).[70]

adoption and not to termination of parental rights, Kentucky surrogate agencies contend that they can pay surrogates who simply relinquish their parental rights, the child thereafter going to its father.* Kentucky's attorney general, Steven Beshear, however, disagrees, noting that the statutory intent in both instances is to give the mother time to think it over. He has written an opinion that surrogate contracts are illegal and unenforceable in Kentucky and has filed suit against Surrogate Parenting Associates, Inc., to enjoin them from continuing their business in the state.[109–112]

The Michigan courts are the only ones to have ruled on the question directly. In a suit filed by Noel Keane to declare unconstitutional those sections of the Michigan Adoption Code that prohibit the payment of surrogates in connection with adoptions, the court ruled that the statutes were valid. It held that they did not prohibit the couple from having a child, but only from "paying consideration in conjunction with their use of the state's adoption procedures" (p. 164).[113]† Reasonable arguments can be advanced in favor of paying surrogates for ovum donation and womb rental or uterine services.[116] Nevertheless, we do not believe it is in the public interest to encourage payment for these services by changing the law because, even though services are being purchased, what is really wanted and, for all practical purposes, what is principally being purchased is a child.[117] That is the *only* reason such contracts are entered into and the only reason payment is made.

While economists may argue the benefits of baby selling and probably of slavery, their arguments generally remind one of the old definition of an economist—someone who knows the price of everything and the value of nothing.[118,119] We see no reason to forbid a woman (a relative or friend) from deciding to bear a child for another woman out of compassion or love; but payment for such a service could encourage the view that children are commodities, and since this would likely be harmful to children, payment should continue to be forbidden.

IVF with a surrogate involves at least one other major issue—who is the mother? We believe that the current legal assumption should remain, any contract to the contrary notwithstanding, i.e., the womb

---

* See, for example, the interview with Richard Levin of Louisville, Kentucky's Surrogate Parenting Associates, Inc.[108]

† The case is discussed with disapproval elsewhere.[114] However, this case affirmed *Doe v. Kelley,* in which the court had said, "Mercenary considerations used to create a parent-child relationship and its impact upon the family unit strike at the very foundation of human society and is potently and necessarily injurious to the community" (p. 3011).[115]

mother should continue to be considered the natural mother of the child. This arrangement not only provides for certainty of identification at the time of birth (a protection for both the mother and the child), but also recognizes the biological fact that the womb mother has contributed more than the genetic mother to the child and, therefore, has a greater interest in it. This fact has led commentators such as Isaac Asimov to suggest that IVF surrogacy is not likely to be very popular.

> A baby is not, after all, a matter of genes only. A great deal of its development in the fetal stage depends upon the maternal environment; upon the diet of the host-mother, the efficiency of her placenta, the biochemical details of her cells and bloodstream. The biological mother may not feel that the baby she receives from someone else's womb is truly hers, and when flaws and shortcomings (real or imagined) show up in the infant, the biological mother may not patiently and lovingly endure them, but may blame them on the host mother [p. 352].[14]

Whether or not Asimov's prediction is correct, we believe that at present the evidence suggests that surrogate mother agreements are not in the best interests of either the child or society and should be discouraged by both physicians and lawyers. Although we do not recommend legislation to prohibit surrogacy or any other form of human sexual reproduction, all legislative and regulatory proposals should be strictly examined to ensure that their primary thrust is to protect the unrepresented third party involved—the would-be child.

Summary

IVF and ET are remarkable medical achievements that promise offspring to couples for whom it was previously impossible. But these medical procedures raise serious social issues regarding indications, selection, consent, donor oocytes, donor embryos, and surrogate childbearers. Caution and prudence are demanded. Professional standards regarding research in IVF are laudable and should continue to be developed. Public discussion should be encouraged. Donor embryos and surrogate childbearing for IVF should, at least at this time, be discouraged. Too many potential problems exist for too little potential benefit. Model legislation seems premature, although it certainly is time to sharpen the issues and determine what steps we can take to protect the would-be children and society itself from the negative potentials of IVF and ET.

In Orwell's *1984,* "The Ministry of Peace concerns itself with War, the Ministry of Truth with lies, the Ministry of Love with torture, and the Ministry of Plenty with starvation" (p. 178).[10] It is similar double-think to believe that anything goes if the goal is to produce a child for an adult who wants one. As Aldous Huxley wrote more than twenty-five years after he imagined *Brave New World*:

> *Brave New World* presents a fanciful and somewhat ribald picture of a society in which the attempt to recreate human beings in the likeness of termites has been pushed almost to the limits of the possible. That we are being propelled in the direction of *Brave New World* is obvious. But no less obvious is the fact that we can, if we so desire, refuse to cooperate with the blind forces that are propelling us [pp. 24–25].[12]

References

1. Hollister, A. Test-tube baby boom: small miracles of love and science. Life, November 1982, pp 44–52.
2. Ethics Advisory Board, Department of Health, Education, and Welfare. Report and conclusions: HEW support of research involving human in vitro fertilization and embryo transfer. Washington, DC: US Government Printing Office, 1979.
3. Keane, N and Breo, D. The surrogate mother. New York: Everest House, 1981.
4. Medical Research Council. Research related to human fertilization and embryology. Br Med J 285:1480, 1982.
5. Levine, C. In Britain and Australia, new in vitro guidelines. Hastings Ctr Rprt 132:2, 1983.
6. Duncan. BMA proposes guidance over in vitro fertilization. Pulse 43:1, 1983.
7. Grobstein, C. From chance to purpose: an appraisal of external human fertilization. Reading, MA: Addison-Wesley, 1981.
8. Culliton, B. Gore proposes oversight of genetic engineering. Science 218:1098, 1982.
9. Drinan, R. Family law in the twenty-first century. Presented to Family Law Section, American Bar Association annual meeting, San Francisco, 1982.
10. Orwell, G. 1984. New York: New American Library, 1949.
11. Huxley, A. Brave new world. New York: Harper and Row, 1931.
12. Huxley, A. Brave new world revisited. New York: Harper and Row, 1958.
13. Zamiatin, E. We. 1924.
14. Asimov, I. A choice of catastrophies. 1979.
15. Shenk, SL. Das saugethierei kunstlich befruchet arisserhalb des mutterthieres. Mitth Embryol Inst K K Univ Wein 107, 1878.
16. Heape, W. Preliminary note on the transplantation and growth of mammalian ova within a uterine foster mother. Proc Royal Soc 48:457, 1890.
17. Austin, C. Observations on the penetration of the sperm into the mammalian egg. Aust J Sci Ser 84:581, 1951.
18. Chang, M. Fertilizing capacity of sperm deposited in the fallopian tube. Nature 168:697, 1951.

19. Thibault, C, Dauzier, L, and Wintenberger, S. Etude cytologique de la fecondation in vitro de loef de la labine. C R Soc Biol 148:789, 1959.
20. Chang, M. Fertilization of rabbit ova in vitro. Nature 184:466, 1959.
21. Mills, J, Jeitles, G, and Brackett, B. Embryo transfer following in vitro and in vivo fertilization of rabbit ova. Fertil Steril 24:602, 1973.
22. Edwards, R, Bavister, B, and Steptoe, P. Early stages of fertilization in vitro of human oocytes matured in vitro. Nature 221:632, 1969.
23. Steptoe, P and Edwards, R. Laparoscopic recovery of preovulatory human oocytes after priming of ovaries with gonadotropins. Lancet 1:683, 1970.
24. Steptoe, P, Edwards, R, and Purdy, J. Human blastocysts grown in culture. Nature 229:132, 1971.
25. Steptoe, P and Edwards, R. Reimplantation of a human embryo with subsequent tubal pregnancy. Lancet 1:880, 1976.
26. Steptoe, P and Edwards, R. Birth after the reimplantation of a human embryo. Lancet 2:366, 1978.
27. Lopata, A, Johnston, I, Hoult, I, et al. Pregnancy following intrauterine implantation of an embryo obtained by in vitro fertilization of a preovulatory egg. Fertil Steril 33:117, 1980.
28. Jones, H, Jones, G, Andrews, M, et al. The program for in vitro fertilization at Norfolk. Fertil Steril 38:14, 1982.
29. Minneapolis Star, February 19, 1983, p 1.
30. Johnston, I, Lopata, A, Speirs, A, et al. In vitro fertilization: the challenge of the eighties. Fertil Steril 36:699, 1981.
31. DeCrespigny, L, O'Herlihy, C, Robinson, H, et al. Ultrasound in in vitro fertilization. Fertil Steril 35:25, 1981.
32. Testart, J, Frydman, R, Feinstein, M, et al. Interpretation of plasma luteinizing hormone assay for the collection of mature oocytes from women: definition of luteinizing hormone surge-initiating rise. Fertil Steril 36:50, 1981.
33. Seibel, M, Smith, D, Levesque, L, et al. The temporal relationship between luteinizing hormone surge and human oocyte maturation. Am J Obstet Gynecol 142:568, 1982.
34. Mishell, D. In vitro fertilization: state of the art—what can we offer patients? Contemp Ob/Gyn 20:219, 1982.
35. Lopata, A, Johnston, I, Leeton, J, et al. Collection of human oocytes at laparoscopy and laparotomy. Fertil Steril 25:1030, 1974.
36. Trounson, A, Mohr, L, Wood, C, et al. Effect of delayed insemination on in vitro fertilization, culture and transfer of human embryos. J Reprod Fertil 64: 285, 1982.
37. Sathananthan, A and Trounson, A. Ultrastructural observations on cortical granules in human follicular oocytes cultured in vitro. Gamete Res 5:191, 1982.
38. Trounson, A and Wood, C. Extracorporeal fertilization and embryo transfer. Clin Obstet Gynecol 8:681, 1981.
39. Edwards, R, Steptoe, P, and Purdy, J. Establishing full-term human pregnancies using cleaving embryos grown in vitro. Br J Obstet Gynecol 87:737, 1980.
40. Walters, W and Singer, P, eds. Test tube babies. New York: Oxford University Press, 1982.
41. Steptoe, P, Edwards, R, and Purdy, J. Clinical aspects of pregnancies established with cleaving embryos grown in vitro. Br J Obstet Gynecol 87:757, 1980.

42. Wood, C, Trounson, A, Leeton, J, et al. Clinical features of eight pregnancies resulting from in vitro fertilization. Fertil Steril 38:22, 1982.

43. Trounson, A and Conti, A. Research in human in vitro fertilization and embryo transfer. Br Med J 285:244, 1982.

44. Smith, D, Pike, I, Tucker, M, et al. Tubal pregnancy occuring after successful in vitro fertilization and embryo transfer. Fertil Steril 38:105, 1982.

45. Katz, B. Legal implications and regulation of in vitro fertilization. *In* Genetics and the law II, A Milunsky and GJ Annas, eds, pp 351–367. New York: Plenum, 1982.

46. Flannery, D, Weisman, C, Lipsett, C, et al. Test tube babies: legal issues raised by in vitro fertilization. Georgetown Law J 67:1295, 1979.

47. Lorio, K. In vitro fertilization and embryo transfer: fertile areas for litigation. SW Law J 35:973, 1982.

48. The 'brave new baby' and the law: fashioning remedies for the victims of in vitro fertilization. Am J Law Med 4:319, 1978.

49. Lawmaking and science: a practical look at in vitro fertilization and embryo transfer. Detroit College Law Rev 2:429, 1979.

50. Love's labor lost: legal and ethical implications in artificial human procreation. J Urban Law 58:459, 1981.

51. Oakley, M. Test tube babies. Fam Law Q 8:385, 1974.

52. New reproductive technologies: the legal problem and a solution. TN Law Rev 49:303, 1982.

53. Mason, J. Abnormal conception. Aust Law J 56:347, 1982.

54. *Del Zio v. Presbyterian Hospital,* 74 Civ 3588 (SD NY), April 12, 1978.

55. Hubble. Liability of the physician for the defects of a child caused by in vitro fertilization. J Legal Med 2:501, 1981.

56. Palm and Hirsh. Legal implications of artificial conception. Med Trial Techn Q 28:404, 1982.

57. McLaughlin, L. Hub hospitals plan test-tube fertilizations. Boston Globe, March 2, 1983, p 1.

58. Krimmel, H and Foley, M. Abortion: an inspection into the nature of human life and the potential consequences of legalizing its destruction. Univ Cincinnati Law Rev 46:725, 1977.

59. *Smith v. Fahner,* No. 82 C 4324 (ND IL), 1984.

60. *Roe v. Wade,* 410 US 113, 1973; *Maher v. Roe,* 432 US 464, 1977.

61. *Harris v. McRae,* 448 US 297, 1980.

62. *Planned Parenthood v. Danforth,* 428 US 52, 1976.

63. *Bellotti v. Baird,* 443 US 622, 1979.

64. Flaum, J. Slip opinion. *Smith v. Hartigan,* 82 C 4324 (DC IL), February 4, 1983.

65. Grobstein, C. The moral use of spare embryos. Hastings Ctr Rprt 11:5, 1982.

66. Johnston, I. The moral status of the embryo. *In* Test tube babies, W Walters and P Singer, eds, pp 49–63. New York: Oxford University Press, 1982.

67. Shapley, D. New UK row on embryo research. Nature 299:383, 1982.

68. Currie-Cohen, M, Luttree, L, and Shapiro, S. Current practice of artificial insemination by donor in the United States. N Engl J Med 300:585, 1979.

69. Somerville, M. Birth technology, parenting and deviance. Int J Law Psychiatr 5:123, 1982.

70. Tiefel, H. Human in vitro fertilization: a conservative view. JAMA 247:3235, 1982.
71. Annas, GJ. Allocating artificial hearts in the year 2002: *Minerva v. National Health Service.* Am J Law Med 3:59, 1977.
72. Annas, GJ, Glantz, LH, and Katz, BF. Informed consent to human experimentation: the subject's dilemma. Cambridge, MA: Ballinger, 1977.
73. Capron, A. The continuing wrong of wrongful life. *In* Genetics and the law II, A Milunsky and GJ Annas, eds, pp 81–93. New York: Plenum, 1982.
74. Furrow, B. The causes of wrongful life suits: remunerations on the diffusion of medical technologies. Law Med Health Care 10:11, 1982.
75. Taub, S. Wrongful life: its problems are not just semantic. Law Med Health Care 10:208, 1982.
76. Annas, GJ. Righting the wrong of wrongful life. Hastings Ctr Rprt 11:8, 1981.
77. Partridge, E, ed. Responsibilities to future generations. Buffalo, NY: Prometheus Books, 1981.
78. Trounson, A. Phys Washington Rprt 6:5, December 1982.
79. Annas, GJ. AID: beyond the best interests of the sperm donor. Fam Law Q 14:1, 1980.
80. Trounson, A, Leeton, J, Wood, C, et al. Successful human pregnancies by in vitro fertilization and embryo transfer. Science 212:681, 1981.
81. Craft, I and Yovich, J. Implications of embryo transfer. Lancet 2:642, 1979.
82. Kass, L. Making babies—the new biology and the old morality. Public Interest 26:18, 1972.
83. Kass, L. Ethical issues in human in vitro fertilization, embryo culture and research, and embryo transfer. *In* Report and conclusions: HEW support of research involving human in vitro fertilization and embryo transfer, Ethics Advisory Board, DHEW, appendix. Washington, DC: US Government Printing Office, 1979.
84. Ramsey, P. Fabricated man. New Haven: Yale University Press, 1970.
85. Advertising Age, May 14, 1979, p 30.
86. Elias, S and Simpson, JL. Evaluation and clinical management of patients at apparent increased risk for spontaneous abortions. *In* Embryonic and fetal death, IH Porter and EB Hook, eds, p 331. New York: Academic Press, 1980.
87. Willadeen, S. A method for culture of micromanipulated sheep embryos and its use to produce monozygotic twins. Nature 277:298, 1979.
88. President's Commission for the Study of Ethical Problems in Medicine and Biomedical and Behavioral Research. Splicing life: the social and ethical issues of genetic engineering with human beings. Washington, DC: US Government Printing Office, 1982.
89. Motulsky, A. Impact of genetic manipulation on society and medicine. Science 219:135, 1983.
90. Newsweek, February 14, 1983, p 76.
91. Boston Globe, February 3, 1983, p 3.
92. Rosenblatt, R. The baby in the factory. Time, February 14, 1983, p 90.
93. National Law Journal, January 17, 1983, p 3.
94. Surrogate mother-to-be fights to keep unborn child. NY Times, March 25, 1981, p A12.

95. Freed, D and Foster, H. Family law in the fifty states: an overview. Fam Law Q 16:289, 1983.
96. Keane, N. Legal problems of surrogate motherhood. So IL Univ Law J 1980: 147, 1980.
97. Martin, L. Legislature gets surrogate parenting measure. Detroit News, February 9, 1983, p 10C.
98. Lansing State Journal, January 25, 1983, p 6A.
99. Detroit Free Press, January 25, 1983, p 12.
100. *Syrkoski v. Appleyard,* 8 FLR 2139 (MI Cir Ct, Wayne Co), November 25, 1981.
101. Surrogate motherhood in California: legislative proposals. San Diego Law Rev 18:341, 1981.
102. Parenthood by proxy: legal implications of surrogate birth. IA Law Rev 67: 385, 1982.
103. Harris, L. Artificial insemination and surrogate motherhood: a nursery full of unresolved questions. Willamette Law Rev 17:913, 1981.
104. Contracts to bear a child. CA Law Rev 66:611, 1978.
105. Surrogate mothers: the legal issues. Am J Law Med 7:323, 1981.
106. Surrogate mother agreements: contemporary legal aspects of a biblical notion. Univ Richmond Law Rev 16:467, 1982.
107. Brophy, K. A surrogate mother contract to bear a child. J Fam Law 20:263, 1981–82.
108. Alsofrom, J. Physician sees no problems in surrogate mother business. Am Med News, June 20, 1980, p 3.
109. Kentucky AG Opinion 81-18, January 26, 1981.
110. Kentucky attorney general calls surrogate motherhood illegal. NY Times, January 26, 1981, p C9.
111. Ohio AG Opinion 83-001, January 3, 1983.
112. In defense of surrogate parenting: a critical analysis of the recent Kentucky experience. KY Law J 69:877, 1980–81.
113. *Doe v. Attorney General,* 106 Mich App 169, 174, 1981.
114. Surrogate motherhood: the outer limits of protected conduct. Detroit College Law Rev 4:1131, 1981.
115. *Doe v. Kelley,* 6 FLR 3011, 1980.
116. Dickens, B. The ectogenetic human being: a problem child of our time. Univ W Ontario Law Rev 18:241, 1979–80.
117. Annas, GJ. Contracts to bear a child: compassion or commercialism. Hastings Ctr Rprt 11:23, 1981.
118. Landes and Posner. The economics of the baby shortage. J Leg Studies 7:323, 1978.
119. Podolski, A. Abolishing baby buying limiting independent adoption placement. Fam Law Q 9:547, 1975.

Chapter 20

Resolving the Crisis:
Where Do We Go from Here?
Daniel K. Roberts

The contributors to this volume have traced the malpractice dilemma from its beginnings through the crisis of the mid-1970s to the current urgent situation. They have explained the legal system, defined the players, identified many of the problems, and presented guidelines for management. Nevertheless, the situation grows more desperate as the costs to the system rapidly approach levels that are unacceptable to both medicine and society itself. No one wants the system to self-destruct; therefore, as the costs become increasingly unacceptable, society will begin to demand that a solution be found.

Until that occurs, we physicians must attend to those elements over which we have control and influence. We must continue to practice good medicine and stay current through journals and seminars. We must concentrate on developing and maintaining rapport with our patients, on enhancing our communication skills, and on removing whatever barriers there are to understanding. We must learn about the legal system, its rules and procedures, and how it can assist us, as well as about lawyers, their "tricks of the trade," and how they think.

From our own ranks, those who choose to be experts must learn to evaluate claims completely, objectively, and fairly—a most difficult task in the clear light and casual time frame of retrospect. These individuals must be taught the meaning of *standard of care* and *causation.*

In addition, short of meddling in any given case, we must find ways to combat the big business that has created a community of *medical expert whores* who will "opine, under oath, that the standard of care was something other than what the defendant followed" (p. 217).[1] I cannot help but question the ethics of some of those physicians who advertise for the attorneys' dollars. Here are some sample advertisements from a recent issue of a magazine for trial lawyers.[2]

> We help attorneys win medical malpractice cases . . . . There is no charge or obligation until we have a supportive report from a qualifiable expert [p. 78].

> The right expert witness can make all the difference in your next medical malpractice case . . . . Specialized areas include medical and dental malpractice, hospital negligence, personal injury, workers' compensation, product liability and equipment failure cases. An evaluation for merit service is also available [p.85].

> OB/GYN Expert. Board-certified, FACS, 15 years practice & trial experience, superior credentials, university appointment, ethical approach to medical liability. Will evaluate, testify, travel [p. 90].

The only way to combat such a complex and sensitive problem may well be to eliminate the need for such experts in the adversary system. One solution being explored is to have the court appoint expert medical witnesses or a panel of such experts who would inform the judge and jury in the interests of communication and understanding rather than partisanship and advocacy. Another solution is to replace the present fault-based system. However, until a new system is in place, experts who testify for the defense must be as cunning and skilled as those who sell themselves to the plaintiffs' attorneys.

Another aspect over which we physicians have control and which has been mentioned frequently throughout this book is the role that medical records play in the malpractice problem. In my experience, greater than seventy percent of all malpractice lawsuits are significantly impacted by poor medical records. Complete, timely records make it extremely difficult for negligence to be manufactured.

Physicians once thought that countersuits might deter the plaintiff's bar from bringing frivolous lawsuits. However, since the plaintiff's attorney owes no responsibility to the defendant, almost all have been lost or later reversed at the appellate level. Whether countersuits against the plaintiffs themselves would be successful is uncertain; but, even so, their overall impact would be minimal.

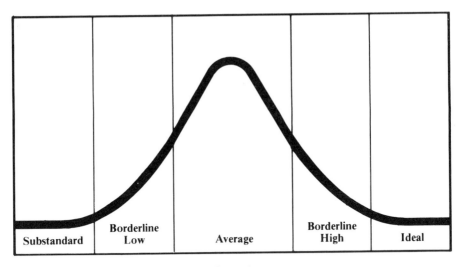

| Substandard | Borderline Low | Average | Borderline High | Ideal |

Figure 1
Standard of Care

Most physicians believe that reforming the tort system itself has little chance of affecting the malpractice problem. The adversary system is based on "what the ignorant ignorantly shall decide to be ignorance" (p. xxiii).[3] We physicians are not being judged by a group of our peers. The system demands that a jury take a gray area and make it black and white. After listening to two equally qualified experts give opposite opinions about what the standard of care required, the jury must decide which one is more believable. There is no allowance for the truth that falls somewhere in between these extremes along the bell-shaped curve of the standard of care (see Figure 1). Sometimes there is no allowance for the truth at all as some juries, in a knee-jerk response of sympathy, award huge amounts to brain-damaged infants regardless of the facts. The jury can relate to the injured plaintiff; they cannot relate to the physician, whose actions are the result of years of training, experience, and education. Because

> jurors do not practice medicine . . . [they] tend to look upon medical matters as a mysterious science. When the results of medical treatment are poor, the jury relates only to an ill or infirm plaintiff, with only a limited understanding of the defendant health care provider's actions [p. 331].[4]

Juries and patients both labor under the same insensitivities to the dilemmas and demands faced by busy physicians, the same misconceptions about the realistic expectations of an imperfect science, and the same misunderstandings about the relationship between incredibly high awards and the increasing health care costs that must be paid by everyone.

Proposals for Resolution

Medical malpractice is no longer an *issue* or a *problem*. It is a *crisis*. Scholars and practitioners from each of the vested interests—physicians, patients, attorneys, and insurance carriers—are moving beyond the complaining stage and are beginning to explore the causes of the crisis and to offer solutions. Perhaps as the adversarial relationship of the vested interests changes to a cooperative spirit, equitable solutions will be found. Of the proposals being thrown into the ring for consideration, each has eloquent proponents, each has positive aspects, and each has serious flaws.

Modification of the tort system has already been attempted with questionable success. In response to the crisis of the mid-1970s, many state legislatures passed measures to readjust a tort system that was decidedly pro-plaintiff. In anticipation that awards would be lower because of the publicity surrounding the earlier crisis, there was a lull in malpractice lawsuits filed in the late 1970s. However, the effects of the legislative measures were only temporary as evidenced by the increasing frequency and severity of claims and an even more liberal judicial environment. In fact, one study found that only two such attempts—total award limitation and modification of the collateral source rule—had slightly measurable influence.[5] Although modifying the collateral source rule may withstand appellate court review, its impact is much less than total award limitation. However, legislation limiting the total award rarely withstands a constitutionality test at the state supreme court level.

In an attempt to bypass this constitutionality problem, Florida physicians attempted to put before the voters a constitutional amendment to limit awards; however, the voters were not allowed to voice an opinion on the measure because it was removed from the ballot on a technicality. Such a remedy could have a very real impact on the costs related to malpractice litigation and an appropriately structured referendum may be worth exploring.

Even those who would preserve the tort system offer proposals to reform its lack of predictability and fairness. Two such suggestions for reform are:

- Damage awards should be structured to resemble the insurance people buy voluntarily. Payment for economic loss should follow a schedule based on age and injury severity, not determined on a case-by-case basis. Collateral insurers should have full subrogation rights. Payment for pain and suffering should be eliminated, except in cases of permanently disabling injury, and then should be a modest, fixed amount. Payment should be made periodically, but the amount should be determined at time of trial, to preserve incentives for rehabilitation. An uninsurable fine in cases of gross negligence should replace punitive damage awards.
- The statute of limitations should be relatively short, running from the time of the injury, not from its discovery. The standard of care should recognize different standards for alternative delivery systems and should recognize costs as a defense.[6]

Earlier legislative attempts to reform the tort system have produced barely measurable success. Not wanting to repeat the mistakes of the past, I question whether or not these measures, once removed from the realm of theory, could have a modest impact, let alone any significant effect, on a situation that is out of control.

Another proposal that appears to be gathering growing interest is removing malpractice actions from the tort system and adopting a no-fault patient compensation mechanism. Advocates for abandoning the fault-based tort system in medical malpractice cases present persuasive arguments based on the notion that the tort system is an unpredictable lottery.

- Determining fault is one unpredictable aspect of the present system. Both plaintiffs and defendants roll the dice when judges and juries are asked to assign fault by unraveling "the often largely unknown mysteries of causation of injury and illness and to determine the appropriateness of treatment procedures about which even experts are often bitterly divided."[7]
- The process is lengthy, with many cases taking eight years or more to be resolved. In fact, the present system rewards delay since prolonged litigation wears down the parties and since inflation makes tomorrow's dollars cheaper than today's dollars.
- Compensation is awarded erratically. Some injured patients receive nothing at all. Some patients receive windfall awards for expenses already paid for by collateral sources. Awards for non-economic damages, such as loss of consortium and pain and suffering, are completely subjective items that are based solely upon highly emotional appeals to the jury's sympathy.

- Transaction costs are enormous. Injured patients receive only 28¢ out of each dollar spent on malpractice insurance.[8] The other 72¢ is the price that society pays for operating this unsatisfactory lottery.

The California Medical Insurance Feasibility Study provided basic data on just how many patients suffered injuries that were potentially compensable in 1974.[9] Because these data indicate that compensating all those with potentially compensable injuries would bankrupt any patient compensation system, proponents of no fault have been ignored until recently. However, the increases in frequency of claims, amounts of awards, attorney fees, and the overall cost of litigation not only demand a reevaluation of the various no-fault proposals but also underline the need for more recent data.

Three pure no-fault systems already exist and could provide models for investigation. There is one in New Zealand, another in Sweden, and the third is right here in the United States—workmans' compensation. Adopting a program where fault and therefore negligence is not at issue would require both parties to compromise. Health care providers would give up the immunity they have for instances when they are not at fault, and patients would give up the possibility of a huge award. In exchange, health care providers would accept the immunity from those injuries that are their fault, and patients would accept smaller, but sure and prompt compensation. Such a program addresses the many shortcomings of the present fault-based system of civil law and recognizes that compensable injuries, maloccurrences, and imperfect outcomes are some of the costs of advancing technological medicine.

Federal legislation proposing a modified no-fault solution was introduced in 1984. The Alternative Medical Liability Act (HR 5400) would give both providers and patients the option to avoid the tort lottery.[10] Providers in federally funded programs could gain immunity from potential liability for noneconomic damages by assuming responsibility for acts of malpractice through offering to pay a patient's economic losses, i.e., out-of-pocket expenses plus reasonable attorney fees. If the provider tenders such an offer, the patient who accepts it loses his ability to sue for noneconomic damages. The patient who chooses not to accept the tender can pursue his claim through the tort system, but cannot include economic losses in the suit, i.e., he can only sue for noneconomic damages. Although HR 5400 has many drawbacks, it does indicate that society is beginning to express its concern about health care costs and that politicians are beginning to respond by seeking solutions.

Other solutions are coming from those who examine the impact of market forces, such as the new consumerism among patients and the competition that created alternative health care delivery systems. They are looking beyond legislative reforms to the legal area of contracts.

> Whereas legislative proposals typically involve cutting back on patients' legal rights, contracts in which consumers surrender those same rights voluntarily are feasible only when providers offer concessions [and alternatives] that consumers perceive to be a fair exchange.[11]

Heretofore, contracts limiting liability for medical malpractice between individuals and their doctors have been struck down as being one-sided. However, when two equal entities, e.g., a labor union and a health maintenance organization (HMO), contractually agree to give up something in order to get something else, the parties would no longer be considered unequal, and the contract valid. For example, the labor union, bargaining on behalf of its members, would agree to submit all malpractice claims to binding arbitration; the HMO would agree to offer lower prices. Those who argue for contractually changing providers' responsibilities and patients' rights believe that people, if given the choice, would choose to lower the standard of care in exchange for lower costs.

Conclusion

From all quarters the suggestions come, but the question remains—where do we go from here? There is, of course, no one answer. For physicians to attack on several different fronts simultaneously seems to offer the greatest likelihood of success. I have identified four such fronts that hold some promise: improving the defense of court cases; educating physicians about risk management; supporting appropriate political and legislative reforms; and contributing time and talent to informing the public about their stake in this crisis.

But before we jump on the bandwagon of any particular solution, I think that we as individuals and we as a society must approach the crisis logically so that we do not repeat the mistakes already made. We need to answer personally as well as collectively some of the following questions:

- How do I define the malpractice crisis? Is it an economic crisis? A psychological crisis? A social crisis?
- What do I want to accomplish vis-à-vis the crisis? What are my specific goals? What results do I want?

- What methods, strategies, and programs will achieve the results I want?
- What actions can I take or encourage that will accomplish my goals?

Perhaps I might be so bold as to suggest that this book may help you find some answers and encourage you to actively confront the malpractice crisis.

Even though the future holds a glimmer of promise, the current climate is bleak. However, I am convinced that society always eventually cycles to the betterment of all. As the malpractice crisis deepens, as the cost becomes prohibitive, and as the public becomes educated about the destructive effects of maintaining the present system, society will demand a solution.

References

1. Falk, A and Cohn, A. Refining the standard of care—a medicolegal imperative. Med Trial Techn Q 29:214, 1982.
2. Trial 20(10):78, 85, 90, 1984.
3. Stryker, LP. Courts and doctors. New York: Macmillan, 1932.
4. Stratton, WT. The circle closes. J Kans Med Soc 85:330, 1984.
5. Danzon, PM. The frequency and severity of medical malpractice claims. Santa Monica, CA: Rand Corporation, 1983.
6. Danzon, PM. Suggested reforms of the fault oriented system—abstract. Presented at Medical malpractice: can the private sector find relief?, Washington, DC, February 21, 1985.
7. O'Connell, J. The case against the current malpractice system—abstract. Presented at Medical malpractice: can the private sector find relief?, Washington, DC, February 21, 1985.
8. Kansas Medical Society. The malpractice system is out of control. Topeka, KS: Author, 1984.
9. Mills, DH, ed. Report on the medical insurance feasibility study. San Francisco: California Medical Association, 1977.
10. Moore, WH and Gephardt, RA. The alternative medical liability act. HR 5400, April 1984.
11. Havighurst, CC. The market and policy environment for private reforms— abstract. Presented at Medical malpractice: can the private sector find relief?, Washington, DC, February 21, 1985.

Appendixes

Appendix A

Summary of
National Association
of Insurance Commissioners' Study

Charles M. Jacobs

The National Association of Insurance Commissioners' (NAIC) study is a comprehensive analysis of closed medical malpractice claims that were made against physicians, hospitals, and other health care personnel.[1] The data were obtained from insurers whose premiums from medical malpractice insurance had totaled $1 million or more in any year since 1970, and were based on files closed between July 1, 1975 and December 31, 1978. In that forty-two month period, these insurers reported a total of 71,782 closed claims; approximately forty percent of these involved payment to claimants. Sixty percent of the claims and seventy-one percent of the dollar value of indemnity were against physicians.

Of the approximately 28,000 paid claims in the NAIC study, thirty-five percent involved improperly performed procedures and an additional fifteen percent were related to anesthesia care, supporting the widely held view that surgeons and anesthesiologists are at high risk for malpractice claims. In fact, insurers place in the highest risk categories those who practice the major surgical subspecialties—orthopedic surgeons, obstetrician-gynecologists, plastic surgeons, head and neck surgeons, cardiovascular and neurosurgeons, as well as their partners in the operating room, anesthesiologists. The most costly claims in the NAIC study were associated with deliveries, with newborns, and with injuries to the nervous system.

Filing a claim that alleges medical malpractice does not mean, of course, that the defendant is liable or even that the case will go to court. The process from filing a claim to final disposition is long and its outcome is uncertain.

About eighteen percent of the total claims closed in 1978 were disposed of by litigation, compared to seven percent in 1975. Over one-half of all settlements in 1978 were reached after a suit was filed or a trial was in progress. Only about one percent of the claims closed in 1978 were resolved by binding arbitration. Contrary to most physicians' beliefs, the defendant-doctor fares best in those cases decided by trial, eighty-nine percent being decided in favor of the defendant in cases closed in 1978. Of cases that go to trial, all defendants won eighty-eight percent of cases closed in 1978, up from approximately eighty percent in 1975.

The monetary value of claims is high, and the highly publicized judgments of $1 million or more lead the public to believe that such amounts are the norm. However, of the claims in the NAIC study filed against physicians, sixty percent of those closed in 1978 involved no indemnity. Of those claims closed in 1978 that did involve payment, fifty-two percent resulted in payments of less than $10,000. Between 1975 and 1978, controlling for inflation, the average indemnity increased forty-two percent; however, indemnity for claims involving economic loss increased eighty-four percent in real terms.

Of those claims against physicians that were paid in 1978, only 2.5 percent were greater than $100,000. This number represents less than one percent of all claims closed in 1978. While the million dollar awards are increasing, they simply and quite clearly do not represent the norm.

The average time for the disposition of claims ending in payment in 1978 had increased to forty-six months from the date of the incident, up from thirty-seven months in 1975. Claims closed in 1978 without payment averaged thirty-eight months to disposition, up from twenty-six months in 1975.

Reference

1. Sowka, MP, ed. Malpractice claims: final compilation: medical malpractice closed claims, 1975–1978. Brookfield, WI: National Association of Insurance Commissioners, 1980.

Appendix B

Summary of
California Medical Insurance
Feasibility Study

Charles M. Jacobs

The data derived from the National Association of Insurance Commissioners' (NAIC) study involved only those disabilities for which insurance claims and lawsuits were filed.[1] The NAIC data, therefore, do not represent the actual incidence of medically caused patient disabilities. The California Medical Insurance Feasibility Study (CMIFS) was an attempt to look beyond the claims filed and to analyze potential claims or patient injuries.[2] One proposed solution to the medical malpractice crisis was to institute a no-fault compensation system, i.e., an injured patient would be compensated for his injury regardless of fault. However, these no-fault proposals suffered from a lack of information about the frequency and severity of medically caused patient disabilities. Without such information, reasonable cost estimates for such schemes could not be made. The CMIFS was an attempt to fill this information gap.

The potential for injuries, liability, and claims discovered by the CMIFS is shown in Figure 1. Box A represents the total incidence of medically caused patient disabilities. Box B represents the incidence of legal fault by members of the health care professions (e.g., carelessness, failure to disclose risks for consent purposes, failure to warn or instruct patients) but which do not result in patient disability. The overlap of Boxes A and B (Area C) constitutes the theoretical incidence of legal liability in our present fault system of litigation, i.e., legal fault is responsible for those medically caused disabilities.

> Most experts and nearly all physicians have assumed that the frequency of fault-caused, patient disabilities (Area C) is substantially less than the total number of medically caused disabilities (Box A), most of which are not the result of legal misconduct. But until the present Study, no one has had sufficient data from which to make reasonable estimates [p. 2].

The CMIFS adopted the following terms and definitions in its analysis. A *potentially compensable event* (PCE) is a disability caused by health care management. A *disability* is a temporary or permanent impairment of physical or mental function, including disfigurement, or economic loss in the absence of such impairment. *Causation* is established when the disability is more probably than not attributable to health care management. Finally, *health care management* includes

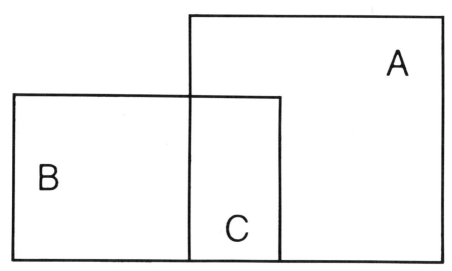

Figure 1*

Potential Injuries, Liability, and Claims

---

* Reprinted with permission (p. 2).[2]

both the affirmative actions (commission) and inactions (omission) of any health care provider or attendant, whether or not such actions or inactions constitute legal fault.

The three classes of PCEs that were measured in the CMIFS are described below, although other types of PCEs may also occur:

Class 1: *Adverse Effects of Treatment.*
This classification includes the adverse effects of commission in health care management, i.e., the occurrence of a new abnormal condition caused by a treatment or procedure, either diagnostic or therapeutic. This type of disability or injury is the one most commonly associated with malpractice litigation, e.g., a severed ureter during hysterectomy, recurrent laryngeal nerve damage during thyroidectomy, and drug reactions.

Class 2: *Effects of Incomplete Diagnosis or Treatment.*
This class involves the failure to realize an expected outcome through acts of commission or omission in health care management, i.e., the occurrence of a discrepancy between expected and demonstrated outcomes of an original abnormal condition for which health care management was sought or rendered. Thus, when a patient's original disease or condition persists, gets worse, or recurs because of a delay in diagnosis or a delay in treatment, there is a discrepancy between expected and demonstrated outcome. Examples include cancer metastasis resulting from a medical delay in diagnosing and treating the original lesion and prolonged postoperative disability arising from the preoperative rupture of an appendix that resulted from a medical delay in diagnosis or a surgical delay in the treatment of an otherwise uncomplicated acute appendicitis.

Class 3: *Effects of Incomplete Prevention or Protection.*
This class includes de novo abnormal conditions that are caused by omissions in health care management, i.e., the occurrence of an abnormal condition caused by incomplete preventive or protective health care management. Examples include the development of a communicable disease caused by lack of prior immunization; an injury caused by falling from a hospital bed; interpersonal disease transmission, such as tuberculosis; the occurrence of a medically contraindicated pregnancy because sexual sterilization or contraception were not recommended; and suicide in the hospital.

A sample of 20,864 records of patients who were hospitalized in California during 1974 were screened against a set of generic criteria. The records that failed to meet the criteria were reviewed by the principal investigators, a team of physician-lawyers experienced in the analysis of medical records. This methodology identified 970 PCEs that were deemed discoverable in 1974, or a PCE incidence rate of 4.6 percent of the sample. These PCEs were then classified according to severity (see Table 1). Based on this model, the PCEs discoverable in 1974 were rated and recorded (see Table 2). The principal investigators concluded that malpractice liability would probably have been found

---

Table 1*

Severity of Disability of Potentially Compensable Events

3.0   **Minor Temporary Disability**

Infections, misset fracture, fall in hospital. Disability not requiring surgery. Recovery delayed, but less than thirty days.

3.1   **Minor Temporary Disability**

Disability requiring surgery. Recovery less than thirty days.

3.2   **Major Temporary Disability**

Burns, surgical material left, drug side-effect, brain dysfunction. Recovery delayed, longer than thirty days but less than two years.

3.3   **Minor Permanent Partial Disability**

Loss of fingers, loss or damage of organs. Includes functional, nondisabling injuries.

3.4   **Major Permanent Partial Disability**

Deafness, loss of limb, loss of eye, loss of one kidney or lung. Disability "not sufficient to cause complete loss of the ability to perform most ordinary functions."

3.5   **Major Permanent Total Disability**

Paraplegia, blindness, loss of two limbs, brain damage. Disability "usually sufficient to alter life-style into a dependent position."

3.6   **Grave Permanent Total Disability**

Quadriplegia, severe brain damage, lifelong care, or fatal prognosis.

3.7   **Death**

---

* Modified and reprinted with permission (p. 53).[2]

Table 2*

Grouped Severity Ratings for PCEs Discoverable in 1974

Severity	Occurrences	% of Total
Temporary (3.0–3.2)	776	80.0%
Minor Permanent (3.3)	63	6.5%
Major Permanent (3.4–3.6)	37	3.8%
Death (3.7)	94	9.7%
Totals	970	100.0%

* Reprinted with permission (p. 53).[2]

in 165 or 17 percent of the 970 PCEs if a claim had been filed. They also noted that the higher the nonfatal PCE severity, the greater the probability that the PCE would lead to liability (see Table 3).

Extrapolating this data to all 3,011,000 admissions to nonfederal, short-term general hospitals in California during 1974 suggests that 140,000 PCEs occurred during that year. Of these, 80 percent (112,000) were expected to be only temporary disabilities; another 6.5 percent (9,100) were expected to involve no functional handicaps. Nevertheless, substantial functional disability was expected in 3.8 percent (5,300) of the PCEs. Extrapolation from the sample data also suggests that 25

Table 3†

Proportion of Liability PCEs to All PCEs Discoverable in 1974, by Severity

Severity Code	All PCEs	Liability PCEs	Liability PCEs as Percentage of All PCEs
3.0	347	29	8.4%
3.1	249	30	12.0%
3.2	180	33	18.3%
3.3	63	15	23.8%
3.4	22	8	36.4%
3.5	9	5	55.6%
3.6	6	5	83.3%
3.7 (Death)	94	40	42.6%
Totals	970	165	17.0%

† Reprinted with permission (p. 100).[2]

Figure 2*

Summary of CMIFS Findings

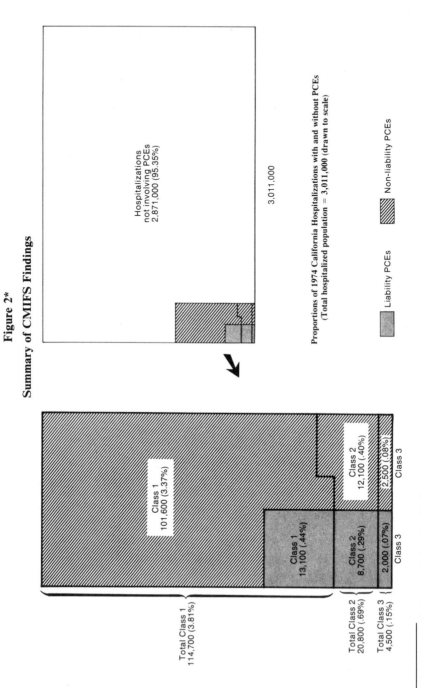

Hospitalizations
not involving PCEs
2,871,000 (95.35%)

3,011,000

Proportions of 1974 California Hospitalizations with and without PCEs
(Total hospitalized population = 3,011,000 (drawn to scale)

Liability PCEs   Non-liability PCEs

Class 1
101,600 (3.37%)

Class 2
12,100 (.40%)

Class 3

2,500 (.08%)

Class 1
13,100 (.44%)

Class 2
8,700 (.29%)

Class 3

2,000 (.07%)

Total Class 1
114,700 (3.81%)

Total Class 2
20,800 (.69%)

Total Class 3
4,500 (.15%)

* Reprinted with permission (p. 106).[2]

Table 4*

Occurrences of Liability PCEs in California in 1974 by Severity of Disability

Severity Code	Occurrences	% of Total	Description
3.0	4,200		
3.1	4,300	55.8%	Temporary
3.2	4,800		
3.3	2,100	9.1%	Minor partial permanent
3.4	1,200	4.9%	Major partial permanent
3.5	700	6.0%	Total permanent
3.6	700		
3.7	5,800†	24.2%	Death
Total	23,800		

* Reprinted with permission (p. 104).[2]

† Diminished to 5,000 if those with probable independent deaths within one year are subtracted.

percent (3,400) of the deaths occurred in patients who would have died anyway from underlying causes within one year. Nevertheless, in California alone, some 23,800 PCEs probably occurred in 1974 (see Table 4). The confidentiality requirements of the study made it impossible to investigate how many of these patients actually sought redress for their injuries.

The CMIFS findings are illustrated in Figure 2.

References

1. Sowka, MP, ed. Malpractice claims: final compilation: medical malpractice closed claims, 1975–1978. Brookfield, WI: National Association of Insurance Commissioners, 1980.
2. Mills, DH, ed. Report on the medical insurance feasibility study. San Francisco: California Medical Association, 1977.

Appendix C

Summary of
American Bar Association's
Commission on Medical Professional
Liability Report

Charles M. Jacobs

In response to the medical malpractice crisis of the mid-1970s, the American Bar Association conducted studies that involved policy analysis and recommendations. Following is a summary of the general conclusions reached by the American Bar Association's Commission on Medical Professional Liability (ABA/CMPL), which issued its report late in 1977.[1]

The ABA/CMPL concluded that the legislative efforts to resolve the medical malpractice crisis and prevent its recurrence were not focused on the complex, underlying causes. Engineered by special interest groups and state officials, most of the changes in tort law and in legal procedures were not aimed at the frequency and severity of claims; those that were either encountered constitutional difficulties or did not affect the price of insurance. However, the ABA/CMPL emphasized that the liability system is conceptually correct as applied to medical claims and should not be abandoned. Real progress in solving the underlying problems will be made only if a variety of efforts are undertaken to refine the options. The most critical include:

1. the reduction of medically caused injuries;
2. the development of new models to resolve malpractice disputes; and
3. implementation of innovative insurance mechanisms, with the emphasis on reform kept at the state level.

In addition, the ABA/CMPL recommended to the ABA's House of Delegates three specific policy statements. The House of Delegates modified one and adopted the other two. The one modified would have originally supported agreements to arbitrate existing or future controversies arising from medical care. The modification eliminated the future aspect, and the House of Delegates endorsed the use of arbitration only where the agreement to arbitrate was entered into after the dispute had arisen.

One of the recommendations adopted by the House of Delegates related to changes in seven areas of tort law. The ABA supported changes:

1. giving patients free access to their medical records;
2. establishing professional expert panels for use in controversies;
3. not allowing voluntary payments to injured parties to be admissible at trial;
4. abolishing the ad damnum clause, the allegation of total dollar amount claimed;
5. allowing the pretrial exchange of experts' reports;
6. permitting itemized verdicts; and
7. leaving the decision about whether to allow prejudgment interest to the jurisdiction.

The third statement adopted by the House of Delegates requested further study of twelve other recommendations for changes in tort law. These included:

1. requiring a notice of intent to sue;
2. clarifying informed consent;
3. clarifying statutes of limitations;
4. requiring a written guarantee of results if such is the basis of suit;
5. clarifying res ipsa loquitur;
6. not limiting dollar recovery to a set amount;

7. reducing recovery by collateral source payments;
8. instructing the jury on nontaxability of damages;
9. disallowing punitive damages;
10. establishing a decreasing maximum schedule for contingency fees;
11. liberalizing the locality rule; and
12. permitting the payment of future damages in periodic installments.

These proposed changes support the assumption that the medical malpractice crisis was a crisis of costs—the cost of larger numbers of claims being filed, the cost of increasingly higher awards, and the cost of increasingly unprofitable insurance. Nothing in the ABA/CMPL analysis or recommendations suggested that the crisis was one of increasing patient injury.

Reference

1. American Bar Association. American Bar Association 1977 report of the commission on medical professional liability. Chicago: Author, 1977.

Appendix D

Summary of
American Bar Association's Fund for Public Education Report

Charles M. Jacobs

Begun in early 1976 and completed about a year later, the study done by the American Bar Association's Fund for Public Education (ABA/FPE) analyzed changes in tort law.[1] In addition, it reviewed the status of alternative mechanisms such as binding arbitration and statutory pretrial review panels.

The ABA/FPE report concluded that most of the tort law changes would have, at most, minor impact on insurance costs. The report listed multiple reasons for that conclusion. For example, procedural changes, such as those requiring pretrial exchange of experts' reports, could not, by their nature, have a major impact on the costs or outcome of medical malpractice cases. Changes dealing with informed consent or with res ipsa loquitur had not appreciably altered appellate case law and, in fact, had not even been at issue in a significant number of cases. Shortening the statute of limitations, while perhaps helpful in dealing with the long tail problem, would not significantly reduce the total number of claims, since ninety-four percent of all claims are reported within three years.

The only tort law change viewed as potentially significant was that repealing the collateral source rule. The ABA/FPE estimated that full application of the repeal could save twenty percent in malpractice award costs. The report, however, noted several problems. First, insurers, reluctant to reduce premiums on the basis of theoretical savings, would require credible statistics, developed over several years of experience, documenting the impact of the repeal. Second, repeal of the rule might be held unconstitutional on equal protection grounds. Third, unless repeal of the rule against introducing collateral sources into evidence was accompanied by a requirement that juries must take into account collateral source payments in determining an award, the expected savings would be problematic.

Another potentially significant change in tort law was that of setting a ceiling on recovery in malpractice cases. While such a change would theoretically decrease costs, as a practical matter the ceilings were set too high for there to be any actuarial difference. Thus, premiums would not be reduced on account of this change.

The ABA/FPE report also analyzed two alternate mechanisms for resolving malpractice disputes—arbitration and pretrial review panels. Basing its conclusions mostly on the results of the Southern California Arbitration Project, the ABA/FPE found that significant cost savings could accrue from a carefully managed, sustained arbitration program. The Southern California Arbitration Project carefully compared eight hospitals participating in an arbitration demonstration with a matched control group of nonparticipating hospitals. It found significant reduction in the number of claims filed (over twenty percent), in total indemnity per claim (over thirty percent), and in defense costs (about fifteen percent). In addition, the project hospitals had closed a significantly higher percentage of claims (about twenty percent) than the control institutions.

Pretrial panels, the ABA/FPE concluded, were an unknown quantity, although the arguments of their proponents appear reasonable. Those arguments, that these mechanisms would promote prompt and reasonable resolution of claims with concomitant savings in indemnity payments and expenses, had yet to be fully tested at the time the report was issued.

Reference

1. American Bar Association Fund for Public Education. American Bar Association fund for public education report concerning legal topics relating to medical malpractice. Washington, DC: US Department of Health, Education, and Welfare, Public Health Service, 1977.

Appendix E

Summary of
Warren-Merritt Study

Charles M. Jacobs

State legislatures responded to the medical malpractice crisis of the mid-1970s by passing legislation that addressed insurance availability and that adjusted the litigation system. The Warren-Merritt study, completed in 1976, examined the initial state legislative responses to the crisis—the legislation passed in 1975.[1] Warren and Merritt reported the "near frantic attempt to stabilize deteriorating medical insurance markets" (p. 3). The first type of legislation established various short-term means of assuring insurance availability, e.g., JUAs, reinsurance exchanges, and physician-owned mutual insurance companies. Because of the variability in subject and complexity, the second type of legislation, adjustments in the tort system, was apparently based less on data and more on blind hunch. Warren and Merritt suggested that if it were clear what parts of the tort system had caused or contributed to the crisis, then tort reform would have been more uniform throughout the states.

The substantive changes in tort law and procedure that were made in 1975 fell into three general categories:

1. holdover—changes already in process that were spurred by the crisis, e.g., Good Samaritan laws;
2. directly related—comprehensive responses that functionally re-

quired civil practice changes, e.g., maximum dollar limits on damage awards; and

3. indirectly related—changes, not functionally required by an overall plan, that were aimed at readjusting the balance between plaintiff and defendant in medical malpractice suits, e.g., statutes of limitations.

Specifically, these legislative adjustments in the substance and procedure of tort law fell into eight areas:

1. The *ad damnum clause* is the portion of the claim, of the pleading, that names the dollar amount being sought. The publicity resulting from being sued for a spectacular amount is particularly upsetting to defendants, who feel that if juries had no knowledge of the amount sued for, they would award more realistic and presumably lower judgments. Elimination or modification of the ad damnum clause was adopted by nine states in 1975.

2. The *statute of limitations,* a rule of procedural law, governs the time within which a lawsuit must be brought. Generally the time limit set by the statute begins to run either when the injury occurs or when the injury is discovered. From the plaintiff's viewpoint, time is required to recover from the injury and to prepare a lawsuit; from the defendant's viewpoint, fairness demands that the time to sue be limited. Because most medical malpractice cases are not brought within a year of the injury, nineteen states made adjustments in their statutes of limitations in 1975.

3. The *collateral source rule,* a rule of procedural law, prevents the introduction of evidence about the amount of compensation for medical injuries the plaintiff has received from sources not named in the lawsuit. For example, evidence about the plaintiff's medical expenses that were paid by health insurance, the lost wages that were paid by disability insurance, and the money received from workers' compensation is inadmissible. Defendants argue that juries award the full value of an injury, e.g., lost wages, medical expenses, etc.; therefore, in cases where collateral payments are received, the injured plaintiff receives a windfall. On the other hand, plaintiffs contend that the defendant should not be allowed to benefit from the plaintiff's foresight in providing for financial protection. In 1975, eight states modified or eliminated the collateral source rule.

4. *Contingency fees* are the common mechanism by which plaintiffs'

attorneys in medical malpractice actions are paid. Under the contingency fee arrangement, the attorney receives a percentage of the award, as high as thirty to fifty percent, if the plaintiff wins; he gets nothing if the plaintiff loses. Defendant-physicians and their insurers claim not only that contingency fees cause claims to be for spectacular amounts but that juries, aware of the arrangement, commonly award additional money since they know much of it will not reach the plaintiff. On the other hand, attorneys defend the contingency fee system on the basis that it enables injured patients to sue who could not otherwise afford it; in addition, it acts to screen out nonmeritorious cases because attorneys are unwilling to spend time on cases that have little chance of recovery. During 1975, nine states enacted limitations on the attorney contingency fee system in medical malpractice cases.

5. *Informed consent,* an amorphous concept in tort law, is not uniformly applied in the various states. In general, "an individual's person is inviolate and cannot be touched without his consent" (p. 282).[2] Surgery, of course, is a rather substantial form of touching, and the patient must give prior consent. The nature of the information that must be transmitted to the patient and the nature and form of the consent required from the patient were legislatively clarified in eight states in 1975.

6. The *burden of proof* rests on the party to the litigation who has the responsibility of presenting the jury with clear and convincing evidence of the particular facts alleged. In most medical malpractice cases, the burden lies with the plaintiff who must prove negligence. However, the doctrine of res ipsa loquitur ("the thing speaks for itself") shifts the burden of proof to the defendant, who must prove the absence of negligence. Because of the inappropriate weight given res ipsa loquitur in medical malpractice cases, four states in 1975 enacted some change in the burden of proof or in res ipsa loquitur.

7. The *standard of care* required of physicians is to exercise that degree of skill and care as others similarly situated, which has in the past meant other physicians in the same locality. For a variety of reasons, including greater uniformity of medical education and ease of communication, the term *locality* has been equated with the nation as a whole, at least for some medical specialties. In 1975, four states reversed this trend to a broader national rule by codifying a narrow locality rule. The theoretical basis for such

action is that a broader spectrum of acceptable medical practice protects legitimate variations in health care, especially since patient outcomes may be influenced by several alternate processes.

8. Continuing a trend that was present before the malpractice insurance crisis, six states passed new *Good Samaritan* laws in 1975. These laws protected physicians from malpractice suits in those instances when they provided care outside traditional treatment settings and where there was no prior physician-patient relationship.

Every state in the United States considered legislation during the two years following the onset of the crisis, and forty-three states passed laws touching on medical malpractice. The changes in tort law, however, did not amount to true tort law reform. Rather they were fine-tuning the existing system, small adjustments in the balance between plaintiff-patients and defendant-doctors. To physicians and insurers, who called the situation a crisis and who saw a litigation system gone haywire, the disparity of legislative responses seemed absurd. However, according to the Warren-Merritt analysis, regardless of whether the tort law changes approached the cause or the cure of the crisis, the steps taken by the states had the desired effect—assuring the availability of insurance and stabilizing medical care.

References

1. Warren, DG and Merritt, R, eds. A legislator's guide to the medical malpractice issue. Washington, DC: Health Policy Center, Graduate School, Georgetown University, 1976.
2. Johnson, BA. An overview of informed consent: majority and minority rules. *In* Legal medicine with special reference to diagnostic imaging, AE James, ed, pp 281–294. Baltimore: Urban and Schwarzenberg, 1980.

Appendix F

Summary of
American College of Obstetricians and Gynecologists' Survey on Professional Liability

Elvoy Raines

The information gathered from the American College of Obstetricians and Gynecologists' (ACOG) Survey on Professional Liability is better understood in the context of recent trends in health care costs in the United States.[1] In 1982, health care expenditures rose to $332 billion, or 10.5 percent of the gross national product (GNP), the highest share in history. The increase was approximately twice the general rate of inflation. Total health care outlay in 1982 worked out to $1,365 per person, about $140 more per person than in 1981. About twenty percent of the total went for physician services; about forty percent went for hospital care.

Also in 1982, physicians, hospitals, and other health care providers and institutions paid over $1.7 billion in medical malpractice insurance premiums, a twelve percent increase over 1981. This increase paralleled the overall increase in health care expenditures for the same period, indicating a similar growth trend.

The 1982 ACOG survey, the first of its kind to my knowledge, examines how the members of one specialty are dealing with the impact of professional liability and the threat of lawsuits. ACOG surveyed practicing obstetricians and gynecologists, those physicians with the greatest familiarity and immediate exposure to the risk of being sued, and discovered that the continuous presence of potential legal liability for unanticipated results or poor outcomes of treatment were likely to be stimulating changes in fees and practice habits. Some of these changes might be considered favorable, the legal threat acting as a positive form of behavior modification resulting in better patient care. However, the majority of changes simply translate into patients being charged more for physician services and being subjected to more diagnostic procedures than are necessary, especially in the current environment of cost consciousness in the health care industry.

Primary medical malpractice insurance coverage for obstetrician-gynecologists now falls in the highest level of rates for physician specialists (see Chart 1). Over thirty percent of obstetrician-gynecologists nationally pay more than $15,000 per year for coverage. But more illuminating and foreboding for the rest of the nation is that in the highly urbanized states—where the professional liability issue for physicians is most fully developed—the percentage of physicians who pay over $15,000 per year is 75.8 percent in New York, 62.6 percent in Florida, and 65.9 percent in California. In the Southeast, excluding Florida, the risk of lawsuit is low. But as the Rand Corporation's national study of medical malpractice claims concluded, this problem is a product of urbanization and, therefore, is a concern for all states as they catch up with their more developed neighbors.[2]

The response of physicians is clear (see Chart 2). About twenty percent of the physicians in New York and almost that many in Florida have increased their fees by more than thirty percent.

Chart 1

Cost of Liability Insurance (Primary Coverage)

	Nation	New York	Florida	California
Less than $8,000	30.8%	7.8%	12.5%	15.9%
$8,000–$15,000	35.5	15.0	24.0	15.8
$15,000–$35,000	30.4	65.6	59.6	63.9
More than $35,000	2.0	10.2	3.0	2.0

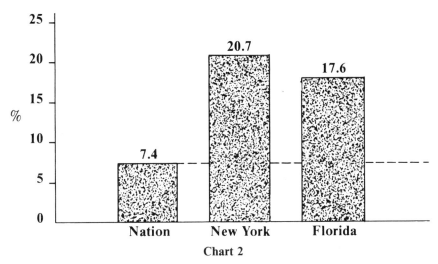

Chart 2

Increase in Fees in Past 2 Years Due to Liability Premiums (30% or More)

While it is fitting to be concerned about health care costs and direct fee increases to patients, our concern grows more significant when this sort of problem inspires changes in the *manner* and *scope* of practice (see Chart 3). The study reveals that while gynecologic surgery is the basis for lawsuits in 41.3 percent of cases, delivery and other obstetric

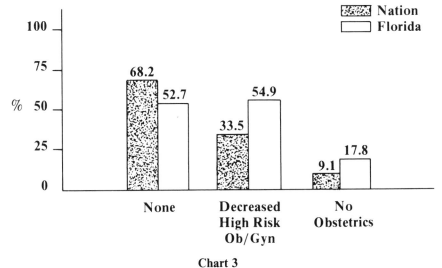

Chart 3

Changes in Practice Due to Malpractice Suits

care account for 49.7 percent of claims. Physicians respond quite predictably—they decrease the amount of high-risk obstetrics that they
practice, or they eliminate their obstetrical practice altogether. In Florida, for instance, while about half of those surveyed did not change the
nature of their practice, half did decrease their involvement in high-
risk obstetrics and gynecology, and 17.8 percent said that they no longer
practice obstetrics.

Obstetrician-gynecologists generally decrease their practice of obstetrics at about age 54; however, this survey shows that due to the
professional liability issue more than a third of those leaving obstetrics
are under 54. This reduction in manpower for the most experienced,
skilled obstetrician-gynecologists is a serious consequence of the medical liability problem.

The frequency of lawsuits leads to changes in practice, not only for
those physicians who have been sued, but also for physicians in general
(see Chart 4). The most frequent changes in practice are increased
testing, documentation, and monitoring of labor. Arguably, obstetrician-gynecologists already conducted an appropriate amount of such
diagnostic and administrative activities; and these increases are per-
fectly understandable reactions to the fear of lawsuits. They drive up

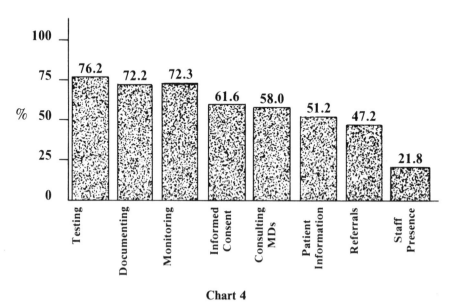

Chart 4

Increased Activities Due to Malpractice Suits

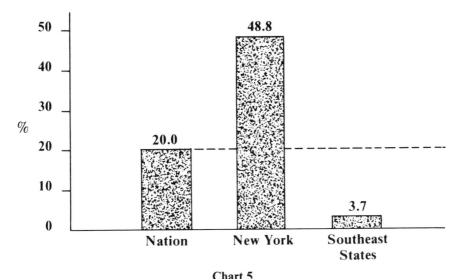

Chart 5
Number of Times Sued (3 or More)

health care costs, as the physicians surveyed recognized, but they are extra precautions that physicians take to eliminate any chance that unanticipated results might occur. Those changes in practice that are considered to be positive improvements—more attention to informed consent, consultation, patient information, and referrals—also contribute significantly to health care costs.

The risk of lawsuit is highest for physicians between the ages of 25 and 44. The more times physicians experience claims or lawsuits, the more likely they are to change their fees and change the nature of their practice (see Chart 5). About 60 percent of the obstetrician-gynecologists in the United States have been sued at least once; and in New York, 48.8 percent of the obstetrician-gynecologists surveyed have been sued three or more times. Of course, lawsuits are frequently dropped, so not that many cases actually go to court. But any claim or lawsuit is costly and contributes to changes in fees and practice. One major commercial insurance carrier spends about $7,000 for legal and administrative costs for claims that are eventually dropped and involve no money payment to the claimant.

The more frequently the physician is sued, the more likely he is to make changes in fees and practice (see Chart 6). As the physician approaches three claims, he is more likely to make some kind of change,

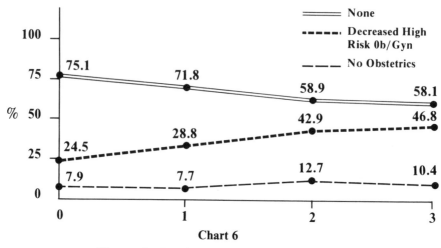

Chart 6

Changes in Practice by Number of Times Sued

more likely to decrease the level of high-risk obstetrics and gynecology, and more likely to retire from obstetrical practice.

Some ask why physicians simply do not "go bare" (practice without insurance) and avoid these costs. That situation does occur. Nationally, about 2.6 percent do not carry coverage, but in Florida that number is more like 5.4 percent and in California, 9.1 percent. Nationally, 10.7 percent have been uninsured at some time; in Florida, 25 percent have been uninsured at some time; and in California, 25.6 percent. Fully 46 percent explain that their reason for being uninsured at some time was their inability to afford the insurance. But the study reveals that they eventually return to buying coverage because they find it too "nerve-racking" to practice without it.

The professional liability problem has grown to such proportions that it is no longer simply a cost of doing business for physicians. It is a major national health policy issue.

References

1. Raines, E. Survey on professional liability. Washington, DC: American College of Obstetricians and Gynecologists, 1983.
2. Danzon, PM. The frequency and severity of medical malpractice claims. Santa Monica, CA: Rand Corporation, 1982.

Glossary of Legal and Insurance Terminology

Abandonment—the unilateral severance by a physician of the professional relationship between himself and the patient without reasonable notice to the patient at a time when there is still the necessity of continuing attention. [*Lee v. Dewbre,* 362 SW2d 900, 902 (Tex Civ App—Amarillo, 1962, No Writ)]

Ad Damnum—"to the damage" part of plaintiff's pleading containing statement of his monetary loss or damages.

Answer—the formal written statement made by a defendant setting forth the grounds of defense.

Apparent Agency—acts by an apparent agent justifying belief in agency, knowledge thereof by apparent principal, and reliance thereon by third party consistent with ordinary care.

Arbitration—use of a third party chosen by the parties to decide a disputed matter.

Assumption of Risk—a defense that applies in situations where the patient has been fully informed of risks incidental to medical diagnosis and treatment, and the patient knowingly and voluntarily agrees to the described procedure. [*Wilson v. Scott,* 412 SW2d 299 (Texas, 1967)]

Best Evidence Rule—in proving the contents of a written instrument, the original instrument must be produced unless the original is unavailable for some reason other than the fault of the party offering the instrument into evidence. [23 Tex Jur 2d, Evidence 209]

Breach of Duty—an omission of a legal duty.

Burden of Proof—the duty of affirmatively proving a fact in dispute. In an action for malpractice, a fact must be proven by a preponderance of the evidence. [45 Tex Jur 2d, Physicians 129]

Captain of the Ship Doctrine—the traditional theory upon which a surgeon has been held vicariously liable for the negligent acts of all those assisting him during an operation. The modern trend is to find liability only where the physician has the right to direct or control the particular details of the work of others. [*Sparger v. Worley Hospital, Inc.,* 547 SW2d 582 (Texas, 1977)]

Captive Insurance Company—owned and controlled by those it insures, as when a hospital, hospital association, or medical society establishes its own medical malpractice insurance company.

Case in Chief—the part of the trial in which the party with the burden of proof presents his evidence.

Case Law—collection of reported cases that form a body of jurisprudence or law from which precedents on a particular subject are drawn.

Claims Made Insurance Policy—covers only those claims made (or notice from the doctor of potential claims that could be made) during the period covered by the policy.

Collateral Source Rule—benefits received by the plaintiff from a source wholly independent of and collateral to the wrongdoer will not diminish the damages otherwise recoverable from the wrongdoer. [*Allman v. Holleman,* 233 Kan 781, 667 P2d 296]

Comparative Negligence—when both the plaintiff and defendant are judged negligent and thus responsible for the plaintiff's injury, their relative negligence is compared, and the award to the plaintiff is reduced in proportion to the amount of his negligence.

Complaint—the first or initial pleading on the part of the plaintiff. Its purpose is to give the defendant information of all material facts on which plaintiff relies to support his demand.

Contributory Negligence—conduct on the part of the plaintiff, contributing as a legal cause to the harm he has suffered, which falls below the standard to which he is required to conform for his own protection. [Second Restatement of Torts, 463]

Counterclaim—a claim alleged by the defendant that is opposed to or deducts from the plaintiff's allegation.

Cross-Claim—one defendant's claim against another defendant in the same action concerning allegations made in the plaintiff's claim.

Damages—the sum of money the law awards as pecuniary compensation for a tortious act. [17 Tex Jur 2d, Damages 1]

> **Compensatory Damages**—an award to compensate the injured party for the injury sustained and nothing more. [Black's Law Dictionary, ed 5, p 352]

> **Punitive Damages**—an award not intended as compensation to the injured person but as punishment to the wrongdoer and as a deterrent to the defendant and others from the future commission of similar offenses and wrongs. [17 Tex Jur 2d, Damages 175]

Deposition—a discovery procedure whereby each party may examine, by oral or written questions, under oath, the other party or any person who may possibly have any knowledge of the subject matter of the lawsuit. [19 Tex Jur 2d, Depositions 1]

Duty—obligation(s) of performance and/or care that conforms to a standard of reasonable conduct.

Evidence—the means by which alleged facts are either proved or disproved. [23 Tex Jur 2d, Evidence 1]

> **Circumstantial Evidence**—proof of collateral facts and circumstances from which it may be concluded that the principal facts at issue actually existed. [23 Tex Jur 2d, Evidence 7]
>
> **Direct Evidence**—proof of facts which tends to show the existence of a fact in question without the intervention of the proof of any other fact. [Black's Law Dictionary, ed 5, p 414]
>
> **Demonstrative Evidence**—the use of articles or objects such as charts and models rather than the statement of witnesses to prove a fact in question. [20 Am Jur 2d, Evidence 497]

Good Samaritan Doctrine—provides a qualified immunity for certain health care providers who administer emergency care gratuitously and in good faith at the scene of an emergency under conditions codified by local statutes.

Hearsay—statements made outside of court by a person other than the one offering the testimony where the witness is merely repeating what others have said. [29 Am Jur 2d, Evidence 497]

Hold-Harmless Agreement—one party agrees to protect another party from loss, i.e., the second party will not suffer any legal harm related to a specific risk it transfers to the first party.

Hostile Witness—may be interrogated by leading questions.

Hypothetical Question—a combination of assumed or proven facts and circumstances, stated in such a form as to constitute a coherent and specific situation or state of facts, upon which the opinion of an expert is asked. [Black's Law Dictionary, ed 5, p 669]

Impeachment—proving a witness is unworthy of belief, usually by showing that the witness has made prior inconsistent statements.

Interrogatories—a discovery procedure in which one party submits written questions to the opposing party, who must respond in writing under oath.

Joint Underwriting Association—an affiliation of insurance carriers that join together to underwrite a particular area of potential loss.

Judicial Notice—the act by which a court accepts as truth the existence of certain facts without the necessity of offering evidence to prove such facts. [23 Tex Jur 2d, Evidence 10]

Leading Question—a question in which the examiner suggests the answer desired from the witness.

Locality Rule—the doctrine establishing that the duty of care owed by a physician to his patient is to be judged by the degree of ability and skill possessed by other physicians in the same or similar circumstances, with his locality of practice merely a factor to be considered. [*Christian v. Jeter,* 445 SW2d 51 (Tex Civ App—Waco, 1969, Ref'd NRE)]

Majority Rule—rule by vote or choice of the majority, i.e., a rule of law in which twenty-six states agree.

Medical Negligence—the acts or omissions of the treating physician, constituting a failure to conform to the standards of skill, care, and diligence required, which results in some injury to the patient. [*Allison v. Blewett,* 348 SW2d 182 (Tex Civ App—Austin, 1961, Reh Den, Err Ref NRE)]

Minority Rule—opposed to majority rule.

Motion for Nonsuit or Directed Verdict—a motion normally made at the close of the party's case by the opposing party asking for a favorable verdict because of a failure of the adversary to establish a prima facie case. [56 Tex Jur, Trial 197]

National Standard of Care—a duty to exercise that degree of care and skill expected of a reasonably competent practitioner in his specialty acting under similar circumstances, and taking into account the advances in the profession. [*Brune v. Belinkoff,* 354 Mass 102, 235 NE2d 793 (1968)]

Negligence—the doing of something that a person of ordinary prudence would not have done under similar circumstances, or the failure to do something that a person of ordinary pruuence would have done under the same or similar circumstances. [40 Tex Jur 2d, Negligence 1]

Occurrence Insurance Policy—covers claims occurring during the period covered by the policy, regardless of when these claims are filed.

Past Recollection Recorded—use of a memorandum, rather than oral testimony, as evidence when the memorandum fails to refresh the recollection of the witness; the witness must testify that the memorandum is a record of the facts when they were fresh in his mind. [23 Tex Jur 2d, Evidence 330]

Physician-Patient Privilege—without the consent of his patient, a treating physician cannot be compelled to disclose information he obtained relative to the treatment rendered the patient. [61 Am Jur 2d, Physicians 169]

Physician-Patient Relationship—arises by contractual agreement, express or implied, and is based upon the dependence of the patient and the learning, skill, and experience of the physician. [45 Tex Jur 2d, Physicians 99]

Pleading—the process performed by the parties to a lawsuit, in alternately presenting written statements of their contention, which serves to narrow the field of controversy.

Present Recollection Refreshed—the use of a memorandum presented to a witness for his inspection which revives his memory and allows him to testify from his recollection and not the memorandum. [23 Tex Jur 2d, Evidence 318]

Prima Facie Case—one that is established by sufficient evidence and can be overthrown only by rebutting evidence adduced on the other side.

Proximate Cause—that which, in natural and continuous sequence, unbroken by any efficient, intervening cause produces the injury. [40 Tex Jur 2d, Negligence 14]

Request for Admissions—statements submitted to an opponent requiring him to admit or deny the truth of some matter alleged by the opposite party.

Request for Physical Examination—a discovery procedure to have a party examined by a physician when that party has put his physical condition at issue in the case. [20 Tex Jur 2d, Discovery 30]

Request for Production—a discovery procedure allowing a party to inspect or photograph designated documents, books, and other tangible items relevant to the matter being litigated, and that are in the possession of the adverse party. [20 Tex Jur 2d, Discovery 17]

Res Ipsa Loquitur—the plaintiff's injury is so clearly the result of the defendant's negligence that "the thing speaks for itself."

Respondeat Superior—the employer is liable in certain cases for the wrongful acts of an employee.

Statute—an act of the legislature declaring, commanding, or prohibiting something. [Black's Law Dictionary, ed 5, p 1264]

Statute of Limitations—statutory law that no suit may be maintained on a claim, unless instituted within a specified period of time after the claim occurred.

Strict Liability—the doctrine finding liability where the defendant's activity is unusual and abnormal in the commmunity, although not necessarily negligent, and the danger which it threatens to others is unduly great and particularly where the danger will be great even though the enterprise is conducted with every possible precaution. [WL Prosser. Law of torts, ed 4, p 494]

Structured Settlement—money paid to an injured party via periodic payments that are fixed and determinable as to amount and time of payment.

Subpoena—the process to cause a witness to appear at court and give testimony.

Summary Judgment—a judgment granted, upon motion, by the court to either party prior to trial where the information disclosed shows that the case lacks a genuine issue with regard to any material fact and that a law applies to those uncontested facts which is favorable to the party seeking the judgment. [45 Tex Jur 2d, Pleadings 131]

Summons—notice to a defendant that a lawsuit has been filed against him and that judgment may automatically go against him if he does not respond.

Tort—an act or omission which unlawfully violates a person's right created by the law, and for which the appropriate remedy is an action for damages by the injured person. [WL Prosser. Law of torts, ed 4, p 2 N 1]

Trial—the judicial examination before the court of the facts put in issue in the case for the purpose of determining the issues. [56 Tex Jur 2d, Trial 1]

Voir Dire—the examination process by which the court and lawyers determine the competency of the jury panel.

Warranty—a verbal or written stipulation that something is or shall be as it is stated or promised to be; a guarantee.

Work Product—no party can require a witness or party to produce or submit for inspection any writing prepared by or under the supervision of an attorney in preparation for trial. [*Alscike v. Miller*, 196 Kan 547, 412 P2d 1007]

Abbreviations

ABA—American Bar Association

ABA/CMPL—American Bar Association's Commission on Medical Professional Liability

ABR—American Board of Radiology

ACOG—American College of Obstetricians and Gynecologists

ACR—American College of Radiology

AID—artificial insemination by donor

ASUTS—American Society of Ultrasound Technical Specialists

CAT—computerized axial tomography

CMIFS—California Medical Insurance Feasibility Study

CNS—central nervous system

CPD—cephalopelvic disproportion

D and C—dilation and curettage

DHEW—Department of Health, Education, and Welfare

EDC—expected date of confinement

EEG—electroencephalogram

ET—embryo transfer

FHT—fetal heart tone

hCG—human chorionic gonadotropins

HEV—hemorrhagic endovasculitis

HSA—Health Systems Agencies

IRB—internal review board

IUGR—intrauterine growth retardation

IVF—in vitro fertilization

JCAH—Joint Commission on the Accreditation of Hospitals

JUA—joint underwriting association

LH—luteinizing hormone

LMP—last menstrual period

L/S—lecithin/sphingomyelin

NAIC—National Association of Insurance Commissioners

NCRPM—National Council on Radiation Protection and Measurements

OA—occiput anterior position

PAC—professional affairs committee

PAP—Papanicolaou's test

PCE—potentially compensable event

PG—prostaglandin

PDR—Physician's Desk Reference

PSRO—Professional Standards Review Organization

QA—quality assurance

QAC—quality assurance committee

RDMS—Registry of Diagnostic Medical Sonographers

RDS—respiratory distress syndrome

SDMS—Society of Diagnostic Medical Sonographers

TORCHS—toxoplasmosis, other, rubella, cytomegalovirus, herpes, syphilis

Index

Mosaic Code of Israelites, 26
mother, surrogate, 231, 234–38
motions at trial, 41–42, 71–73
    definition of, 284
Myers, RE, 149

N

National Association of Insurance Com-
    missioners study (NAIC), 18, 187,
    255–57
National Council on Radiation Protec-
    tion & Measurements (NCRPM),
    202
national health expenditure, 275
National Institutes of Health, 157
national standard of care, definition of,
    284
negligence,
    breach of duty as, 208, 281
    comparative, 161–62, 282
    contributory, 161–62, 282
    damages for. *See* damages
    definition of, 284
    duty &, 30–31, 98, 119, 173–81, 202,
        208–11, 215, 245, 282
    informed consent &. *See* informed
        consent
    law of, 3, 30–31
    obvious, 91–93
    reasonable man standard, 97, 100
    res ipsa loquitur, 91–93
neonatologist-pediatrician, 154–55
New York, malpractice in, 276–80
Nierenberg, G, 106–07
Niswander, KR, 149–50, 152
no-fault compensation system,
    automobile, 13
    HR 5400, 250–51
    medical, 17, 20, 32, 249–51, 257
noninvasive diagnostic tests, 128
nonverbal communication, 87, 105–12
nuclear magnetic resonance imaging, 204
nuclear medicine, 204–05
nurse, 136
    records of, 140, 142

O

O'Brian, WD, Jr., 212
occurrence insurance, 52
    definition of, 284
office practices, 135–39
oocyte, 219fn
    from donor, 231–33
    recovery of, 222–24, 229–30
opening statement to jury, 40, 72
ordinary witness, 41, 79, 81–82
organs, artificial, 230
Orwell, G, 220, 238
ovarian follicle, 223–24
oversight committee, of hospital's board
    of trustees, 194–96
ovum, 219fn
Oxford Cerebral Palsy Study, 152
oxytocic agents, 165

P

Pap smear, 138
past recollection recorded, definition of,
    284
pathologist, 166
pathology specimen,
    abortion &, 130
    Pap smear, 138
    sterilization &, 130
patient,
    as consumer, 47, 115, 123
    attitude of, toward litigation, 4, 10–11,
        17, 19, 46–47
    consent to treatment. *See* consent
    education of, 206–08, 279
    informational needs of, 96–99
    relationship of physician &, 46–47,
        119–20, 126
    selection for in vitro fertilization, 228–
        30
pediatric geneticist, 154–55
pediatric neurologist, 154–55
pediatric records, analysis of, 166–67
peer review, 190, 193
pelvic inflammatory disease (PID), 128,
    138